MENTAL ILLNESS
The Nutrition Connection

How to beat depression, anxiety and schizophrenia

Dr Carl Pfeiffer

ION
PRESS

Acknowledgements

Dr Carl Pfeiffer wished to express his thanks and acknowledge the expert help of Marie Arcaro BA, Elizabeth Jenny MS and Dr Eric Braverman MD. I would also like to thank Tuula Tuormaa, Karen Chung, Graeme Wilson, Kirsten Blaikie and Katherine Monbiot, who, as volunteers for the Mental Health Project have researched and provided material for this book. Our thanks go to all those who have allowed their case histories to be used. A special thanks goes to Suzie, Jan and Heather who have worked behind the scenes, proofing, checking and referencing, and to Dr Abram Hoffer for his help, guidance and lifetime of service for those with mental health problems.

Guide to abbreviated measures

1 gram (g) = 1,000 milligrams (mg) = 1,000,000 micrograms (mcg) Most vitamins are measured in milligrams or micrograms. Vitamins A,D and E are also measured in International Units (iu), a measurement designed to provide standardisation of the different forms of these vitamins that have different potencies.

1 mg of retinol or 2mcg of beta carotene = 3.3iu of vitamin A

1mcg of vitamin D = 40 iu

1mg of vitamin E = approx. 1.5iu of d-alpha tocopherol

References

Many references from respected scientific literature have been referred to in this book. A full list of these references, listed for each chapter, is available from the Institute for Optimum Nutrition, Blades Court, London SW15 2NU. Key references are numbered in the text. Please send £2 and an SAE. Most of these research papers can also be accessed at the Lamberts Library at ION. Please call 0181-877-9993 for details.

Disclaimer

Mental illness is a complex affair. While all the nutrients referred to in this book have minimal toxicity, those seeking help are advised to consult a qualified practitioner who can run the necessary tests and is informed about drug-nutrient interactions. The recommendations given in this book are neither prescriptive, nor should ever countermand the recommendations of your doctor. Neither the author, nor the publisher accept liability for readers who choose to self-supplement.

About the Author

Patrick Holford is widely considered to be a leading international expert on mental health and nutrition. He started his academic career in the field of psychology, researching the role of nutrition in mental illness, while completing his bachelor's degree in Experimental Psychology at the University of York. His fascination with this subject led him to the United States, where he studied the work of Dr Carl Pfeiffer MD PhD at the Brain Bio Center, Dr

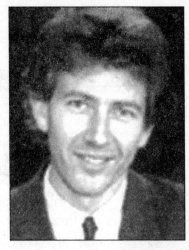

Linus Pauling and other leading figures in nutritional medicine. He has since continued his research into mental health and the importance of nutrients and trace elements such as zinc. In 1984 he founded the Institute for Optimum Nutrition, a charitable and independent educational trust for the furtherance of education and research in nutrition, where he has taught and practised for the past 12 years, as well as lecturing throughout the world. He also directs ION's Mental Health Project and is an International Human Rights Award Winner for his work in this field.

He is one of Britain's leading nutritional authors, writing for a number of major national publications and frequently appearing on radio and television. His books include The Whole Health Manual, Optimum Nutrition, The Optimum Nutrition Workbook, The Better Pregnancy Diet, The Fatburner Diet, The Energy Equation, Supernutrition for a Healthy Heart, How To Protect Yourself from Pollution, Say No to Arthritis and Living Food. He is also editor of Optimum Nutrition magazine.

Contents

Foreword by Dr Abram Hoffer   5

Part 1 - What is Mental Health?

1 Mind over Matter   8
2 Mental Health - The Nutrition Connection   15

Part 2 - Five Steps to Mental Health

3 Food for Thought   20
4 Fats for the Brain   28
5 Brain Pollution   35
6 Beating the Sugar Blues   43
7 Are you a Stimulant Addict?   52
8 Solving the Stress Syndrome   56
9 Brain Allergies   61
10 Smart Nutrients   68

Part 5 - Action Plan for Mental Health

21 Diet & supplements for mental health   196
22 Mental Health & Illness - The Nutrition   74
     Connection

Directory of Supplement Companies   199
Useful Addresses and Recommended Reading   200
Index   202

**See reverse front for Contents of Chapters 11 to 32
on Mental Illness - The Nutrition Connection**

Foreword

I was delighted to read this excellent book written by Patrick Holford and Carl Pfeiffer, deceased. Patrick is a recent friend of mine who will undoubtedly make major contributions to the future of nutritional medicine, judging by his contributions made so far, and Carl Pfeiffer, a long time friend of mine, who was one of the foremost and most productive contributors to orthomolecular theory and practice.

The fist part of this book deals with prevention and the second part with treatment. Both emphasise the enormous importance of developing the correct nutrition for each individual, whether it is for prevention or for treatment. Logically, prevention should come first, and if it were properly and universally applied would much reduce the need for treatment.

As I read this book I was reminded of the long and torturous history that medical nutrition has undergone over the past 100 years. The optimum nutrition for any individual is that which provides the optimum amount and type of nutrients that person must have if s/he is to be normal. For after all, isn't this what nature has been doing for millions of years, fine tuning its creatures to adapt to the available food supply? Linus Pauling knew this and coined the right word, orthomolecular (ortho = right - molecules), to show that the correct amount of natural compounds with which the body is familiar must be used. When we broke away from the basic adaptational rule we began to court major problems.

About 100 years ago food chemists believed that the only component of foods that mattered were carbohydrates, fats and proteins. As a result of this hubris large numbers of the English nobility were destroyed because mothers, instead of using wet nurses, began to feed their babies this pseudo food made up of these three major components. This was the beginning of the first major food experiment which western society willingly adopted. About the same time, the vitamins were discovered, but it was not until the 1930's that the discovery of vitamins flourished. Minerals did not receive much emphasis until about 30 years ago. Dr Carl Pfeiffer was a major contributor to this epoch. This was followed by serious attention to the fats and especially the essential fatty acids, which is only now beginning to flourish.

After one century of exploitation of the public and hurry-up attempts to correct the faults, we are back to the concept that doctors already were aware of many centuries ago, that the best foods are whole foods which contain the fifty nutrients in the proportion nature used.

However, we have made some important discoveries. Since we know the individual nutrients and they are readily available, especially in countries which are more civilised and enlightened, they can be used in optimum amounts which may be large (mega) or small, and which can be individually tailored to suit the needs of the individual, for prevention if they are well, and for treatment if they are ill.

In this book, the information needed to take advantage of the discoveries of the past 100 years is available to intelligent persons, professional or not.

Abram Hoffer MD PhD FRCP(C)

This book is dedicated to creating a future where:

- those with mental health problems have their nutritional status checked, and if necessary corrected
- they can recover in nutritionally oriented half way houses
- psychiatrists realise that a major breakthrough in the treatment of mental illness has occurred, and put it into practice
- and where mental health problems become increasingly rare as society learns how to put prevention into action

If you'd like to help make this happen join ION and participate in the Mental Health Project.

Part 1

WHAT IS MENTAL HEALTH ?

The definition of insanity:
to keep doing the same things and expect
different results.

1

MIND OVER MATTER

One of the extraordinary shortcomings of current thinking is the general denial that psychological phenomenon, such as intelligence or mood, are affected by chemicals, such as food. This is especially strange when you consider that almost every human being has already discovered how to alter their mental and emotional state chemically, by having a coffee, a cigarette or an alcoholic drink (not to mention illegal recreational drugs), and that modern day psychiatry's principle treatment is the prescription of mind-altering drugs.

How we think and feel is not only decided by our social and psychological environment. It is also influenced by what we eat, drink and breathe. The extent by which this is so is only beginning to dawn on us as scientists research new dimensions.

The now famous IQ studies, spawned from the research project of a student of the Institute for Optimum Nutrition, showed that the simple addition of a vitamin and mineral supplement could increase IQ scores by as much as 20 points, with an average increase of at least 4 points in all studies with a duration of three months or more [1]. During the press conference of one of the larger, controlled studies [2], in which Professors Yudkin, Pauling and Eysenck participated, one journalist, referring to those children who had had a 20 point shift in IQ (the average score being 100), asked if this could turn a bricklayer into a brain surgeon. The spokesman affirmed this possibility. An antagonistic journalist pointed out that the average increase was only 4.5 IQ points and asked what this would do. The spokesman said this would turn them into a journalist! Perhaps not the right answer at a press conference, seeking publicity. Yet, the truth is a 4.5 IQ point shift would get many thousands of educationally subnormal children reclassified and returned to 'normal' schools. More comprehensive nutritional programmes have brought severely retarded children, with IQ's in the 40's, back into the normal range [3].

Conversely, the consensus of a wide range of international studies has shown that exposure to levels of lead consistent with the levels found in urban areas where leaded petrol is used, produces an equivalent 4 or 5 IQ point decrease.

But what of you and I? Is there room for improvement in an average adult? The average adult, if such a person exists, used to be the average sub-optimally nourished child, unwittingly exposed to lead. Wouldn't it be inconsistent to find that the mantle of adulthood suddenly protects us from the chemical influences on intelligence?

A New Pair of Glasses

What is needed is a new pair of glasses. A new way of looking at health that takes all factors into account. One that allows us to see psychological and biochemical/physiological processes as interactive, rather than separate. Einstein said that "The significant problems we have created... cannot be solved at the same level of thinking we were at when we created them." So what is this new level of thinking?

Much of today's medicine, and the way we consider our health, is based on the theories of Newton and his contemporaries. They saw the world, and the human body, as a machine. Each part could be broken down and examined to find out how it worked. This thinking, which gave birth to the industrial revolution, led to hospitals with departments for each body system, the idea of transplants and surgical removal of parts that don't work. The concept of 'bugs' causing disease, introduced by Louis Pasteur, added the idea that disease was caused by some outside agent that needed to be destroyed to regain health. Thus we entered the era of a 'drug for a bug' or 'a pill for an ill'. The search for a single cause and a single cure.

Consider the major diseases of today. What's on offer for their eradication? Cancer treatment involves chopping it out, drugging it out, or burning it out with radiation. For heart disease the options include replacing the blocked artery or taking drugs to relax the artery or thin the blood. All very 'mechanical' in concept. For arthritis, there are two kinds of drugs: non-steroidal anti-inflammatory drugs, like aspirin, and steroid drugs, like cortisone. Both kill the pain. Both speed up the progression of arthritis. The same is true for many drugs prescribed for mental illness. They too are pain killers. They don't cure mental illness, and, in many cases, they make matters worse by adding side-effects. These are old ideas based on old ways of thinking that picture an invader (a bug, tumour or blockage) and a defender armed with a weaponry of scalpels, lazers, and chemical weapons. Unfortunately, the medical arms race still continues today. Yet, too often the costs outweigh the benefits. Isn't there a better option?

Any physicist will tell you that Newton is old hat. His ideas were useful to a point, but Einstein's ideas have taken us so much further. So what was Einstein saying and how does this relate to your health?

$E = MC^2$

Instead of viewing life (and disease) as a battle, Einstein believed that everything was not only inter-connected, but made of the same stuff which he called 'energy'. He said that what we perceive as matter (M) is only energy (E) in motion (C). It's like the movies. A film is made of an image, then a space, then an image then a space. But if you roll the film fast enough all you see is a moving image, not the space. If you look at your arm under a microscope it's made out of cells with spaces in between. If you then look at a cell it's made of protein, fat and mainly water. These too are made of smaller units we call atoms, with space in between. The atoms are made of smaller units called electrons, protons and neutrons, with space in between. These electrons, protons and neutrons are made of even smaller particles called quarks, with space in between. In fact, if 'quarks' were real 'matter' the entire matter of the human body would fit onto a pin head! The rest is empty space.

Einstein was saying that everything is the same energy, including the empty space, and that when energy 'condenses' we call it matter. It's a bit 'abstract' isn't it? New ideas are. That's what makes them new. Consider this analogy.

In the old way of thinking cancer is an 'invader' that has to be destroyed. We don't ask so much how it got there as how to get rid of it. In the new way of thinking we see all cells in the body as being manifestations of energy. Normally the energy is directed towards the health of the body. What then happens in a cancer cell? The evidence today points to the idea that cancer cells stop 'talking' to other cells and working for the good of the whole, and instead isolate themselves and become selfish. They enlarge and multiply, develop their own blood supply to get what they need, and start to take over the body like a megalomaniac. What then are the conditions that trigger cells to stop communicating with other cells and working together? This idea of 'connectedness' is inherent in the new model of the universe and in new concepts of health.

Quantum Health

In the new model 'energy' in a system jumps from one level to another. In other words, things change in steps. Ice becomes water, water becomes steam. Our health doesn't gradually, day by day, decline. One day you're well, the next day you're ill. One moment you're happy, the next moment you're depressed. Each step or stage is called a 'quanta', hence quantum physics and quantum health. If you put enough energy into a system it will jump to a higher level. If the system loses energy it will drop to a lower level. So, using our analogy of cancer, the right diet, exercise and frame of mind increase available energy, while the wrong diet, lack of exercise and a negative frame of mind dissipate energy.

This idea of gaining and losing energy is like a 'cost-benefit' equation. Drugs, surgery and radiation all cost the patient energy. So, in these cases the potential 'cure' is itself a promoter of disease. There is a danger here in going round and round in circles. You give a drug to cure one disease, and create another. Then take a drug to counter-act the side-effects of another drug and so on. Many medical scientists are beginning to question if the costs of drugs such as antibiotics, psychotropic and anti-inflammatory drugs outweigh the benefits.

Complex Adaptive Systems

Instead of viewing the body like a machine, modern medicine is beginning to look at us human beings as 'complex adaptive systems', more like a self-organising jungle than a complicated computer. Rather than trying to 'control' a person's health by playing God with hi-tech medicine there's a new way of looking at health that considers a human being as a whole, with an interconnected mind, body and spirit, that is designed to adapt to health if the circumstances are right.

Of course, we are each born different and inherit a different level of resilience or 'adaptive capacity'. So, in this new model, our health is a result of the interaction between our inherited adaptive capacity and our circumstances. For example, on a physical level between our genes and our environment. If our environment is sufficiently hostile (bad diet, pollution, frequent infections, allergies etc.) we exceed our ability to adapt and get sick.

On a psychological level our 'inheritance' is our particular mind frame, the rules we apply to life, based on our upbringing and experiences in the past. Through this pair of glasses we view everything that comes in through our senses, and make our

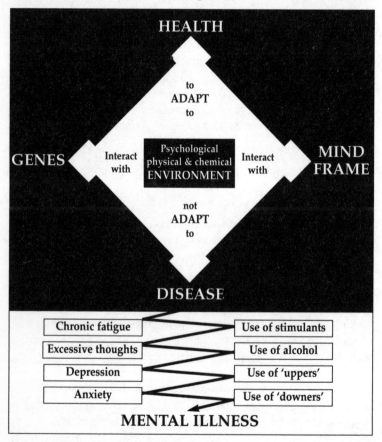

Figure 1 - New Model of Health

judgements. If what we see, hear, smell etc. 'fits' within our mind frame, we adapt to health and maintain psychological equilibrium and health. If it doesn't fit we get upset and lose it.

Einstein spoke about quanta, specific levels that energy manifests in. The psychological equivalent here is the level of our consciousness. The more liberated is our mind frame, or in other words, the less limited is our view of the world, the more we can accommodate the experiences of life, the more we maintain mental health, and indeed, increase it with a greater feeling of well-being and expanded awareness.

Put these two maps - the physical/chemical and the psychological - together and it becomes obvious how one effects the other, as shown in the third map. This shows how biochemical imbalances will affect the mind, and how psychological imbalances will often lead to the use of stimulants and depressants, affecting the brain's biochemistry.

The Amazing Mind

Isn't it amazing that, with all the advances in electronics, nothing comes close to the power of the human mind? Our minds have the capacity to hold trillions of memories. Psychologists estimate that, every day, we have in the region of 60,000 thoughts. And most of them are 'repeats'! Despite all this potential so many people suffer from loss of concentration, memory and mental clarity. More and more children are diagnosed with attention-deficit disorders.

Studies of geniuses and scientists whose insights have changed all of our lives, tend to show that they are not necessarily brighter than other people, but have a developed ability to focus their minds on the question at hand.

We all have amazing mental powers if only we knew how to use them. Most of us dissipate our mental energy by becoming preoccupied with our fears, worries and concerns. We seem to have great 'focus' for our fears, so what would it take to focus all this nervous energy on the task at hand? Many people spend large amounts of time in a state of stress and overwhelm. Nothing depletes vitality more than this. Prolonged stress is associated with an increased risk of 50 physical diseases, as well as depression, irritability and insomnia. Yet, the fact is we create our own stress and overwhelm. They are not caused by outside circumstances, but by how we react to outside circumstances. Sure, changing the circumstances of your life may help, but the most powerful tool at your disposal lies in changing how you deal with situations in your life.

After many years studying mental health I have come to see that good nutrition creates a kind of mental stability and resilience that makes personal transformation more possible. It is as if generating energy from eating the right foods, and simultaneously, not dissipating energy from eating, drinking and smoking energy depleting substances, creates more mental energy or awareness, plus more emotional stability. This, in turn, allows an individual to contemplate issues at a deeper level and move forward. With each step we tap into the seemingly unlimited potential every human being has for insight, expression and for happiness.

2

MENTAL HEALTH - THE NUTRITION CONNECTION

The one major difference between mankind and virtually every other animal is the relatively large size of our brain in relation to body size. Us humans have a brain ten times larger in relation to body size than virtually all animals. There are also chemical differences too, in that our brains have very high concentrations of certain essential nutrients and their derivatives. In fact, during early brain development, no less than half of all nutrients a fetus and young infant receives goes towards brain development.

Scientists have asked why we have these differences and how the brain could have developed in this way. There is now growing evidence that our distant ancestors may have specialised in exploiting a particularly nutrient–rich environment – the water's edge. During early primate evolution we may have lived in swampland and wetlands, eating highly nutritious seafood, shellfish, eggs and vegetation growing in the richest soil, nourished by mineral–rich waters [1]. This optimum nutrition may have provided the raw materials to allow the brains and nervous systems of primates to develop their complexity.

History aside, the fact is that our mental function is totally dependent on a daily basis on receiving a whole host of micro–nutrients, tiny substances like vitamins, minerals and essential fatty acids, that are present in a healthy diet. B vitamins, for example, are needed by every single cell. A long–term deficiency is a known cause of severe mental illness. A short–term deficiency is associated with poor intellectual and behavioural performance. Recently, a series of studies has demonstrated that even adding small amounts of nutrients to the diets of ordinary school children can, for some, have a major effect on their intellectual performance [2].

The basis of 'intelligence' at a chemical level is the communication that goes from cell to cell. Brain cells make 'connections' and in so doing we recognise things, draw analogies and process information. These connections depend on a family of substances called neurotransmitters, which allow information to pass from one cell to another. This is why you remove your hand from fire, as the signal is relayed along nerve cells to the brain, which recognises the danger and sends the message back to withdraw your hand. At every cell intersection neurotransmitters are involved.

Neurotransmitters are made from food. Serotonin, the neurotransmitter that puts you to sleep, is made from the amino acid tryptophan. The body also needs vitamin B3, B6 and iron to produce serotonin. Acetylcholine, the neurotransmitter thought responsible for memory processes, is made from the nutrient choline and pantothenic acid. Your nutrient intake has the power to affect the chemistry of the brain and nervous system, and indeed the whole body, at a fundamental level.

Most drugs currently being used to treat mental illness, as well as recreational drugs used to induce 'altered states', are designed to enhance or block neurotransmitters. Instead of giving drugs, nutrition counsellors often recommend specific nutrients to give the body the raw materials the brain needs to rebalance these neurotransmitters. Such approaches are much safer since these essential nutrients are much less toxic and less expensive than drugs, and are proving to be as

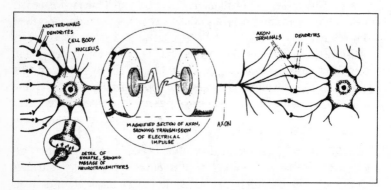

Figure 2 -How brain cells communicate

effective, if not more so, in the treatment of certain kinds of mental health problems.

Even back in the 1960s Drs Hoffer and Osmond were able to demonstrate that so–called schizophrenics could be effectively treated with much larger amounts of vitamin B3 and vitamin C [3]. Dr Carl Pfeiffer at the Princeton Bio Center in New Jersey USA later identified the role of vitamin B6 and the mineral zinc in mental illness [4]. Now we know that deficiencies in magnesium, manganese, B12 and folic acid, as well as zinc and B6 can result in mental illness [5,6,7].

Of course, many people live under the illusion that as long as you eat a well balanced diet you get all the nutrients you need and assume that, however important these nutrients may be, they couldn't possibly be deficient.

Myth of the Well Balanced Diet

The greatest lie in health care today is that "as long as you eat a well balanced diet you get all the nutrients you need". This is a lie because no single piece of research in the last decade has managed to show that people who consider themselves to be eating a well-balanced diet are receiving all the Recommended Daily Amounts (RDA) of vitamins and minerals, let alone those levels of nutrients that are consistent with optimum nutrition. The reality is that the vast majority of us are deficient in a number of essential nutrients, which include vitamins, minerals, essential fatty acids and amino acids, the constituents of protein. Deficient, means 'not efficient', in other words that you are not functioning as efficiently as you could because you have an inadequate intake of one or more nutrients. If this comes as a shock consider the following facts:

• The average person in Britain in 1994, according to the National Food Survey, eats less than the EC RDA of 8 out of 13 nutrients for which RDAs exist. The average intake of zinc is 7.5mg, half the Recommended Daily Allowance of 15mg [8].

• RDA levels vary from country to country. A five-fold variation from country to country is not at all uncommon. In other words scientists don't know what we need.

• RDA's are not optimum. According to the National Academy of

Sciences, who set US RDA's, "RDA's are neither minimal requirements nor necessarily optimal levels of intake" [9]. In the UK, the government funds research to define the optimum intake of vitamins C and E to protect against cancer and heart disease, in recognition of the fact that RDA levels are not necessarily optimum [10]. Factors considered to raise one's requirements considerably above RDA levels include alcohol consumption, smoking, exercise habits, pregnancy, times of stress including puberty and premenstrual phases, pollution, and special dietary habits, for example vegetarianism. Suggested Optimal Nutrient Allowances (SONA's) are often 10 times higher than RDA levels [11].

•There are 45 known essential nutrients. EC RDAs exist for only 13 of these.

•Food does not contain what you think it contains. Most of these surveys are based on recording what people eat and looking up what those foods contain in standard text books. But do they take into account that an orange can contain anything from 180mg of vitamin C to nothing? [12] A 100g serving of spinach can contain from 158mg of iron to 0.1mg depending on where it's grown. Carrots, that reliable source of vitamin A, can provide a massive 18,500ius down to a mere 70ius. Store an orange for two weeks and its vitamin C content will be halved. Boil a vegetable for 20 minutes and 50 % of its B vitamins will be gone[13]. Refine brown flour to make white and 78 % of the zinc, chromium and manganese are lost [14]. Today's food is not a reliable source of vitamins and minerals.

The reality is that many people are deficient in essential brain nutrients and suffer from greater degrees of mental imbalance as a result. A nutritional approach to mental illness involves working out an individual's nutritional status and correcting any potential deficiency with diet and supplements. Much higher levels of nutrients are often needed to restore mental health than are needed to maintain it. There may also be some people who, perhaps for genetic reasons, need higher levels of nutrients than others to maintain mental health.

Part 2

SIX STEPS FOR MENTAL HEALTH

- *Ensure an optimal intake of vitamins, minerals and essential fats.*
- *Detoxify toxic metals and other anti-nutrients.*
- *Avoid sugar, refined foods and stimulants.*
- *Avoid unnecessary stress.*
- *Improve digestion and eliminate allergies.*
- *Ensure an optimal intake of smart nutrients.*

3

FOOD FOR THOUGHT

E very one of the fifty known essential nutrients, with the exception of vitamin D, has a role to play in promoting mental health. Here are some of the key brain nutrients, the symptoms that occur in deficiency, and the best foods to eat, to help you assess if you're getting enough.

The B Vitamins

The B complex group of vitamins are vital for mental health. Deficiency of any one of the eight B vitamins will rapidly affect how you think and feel. This is because they are water soluble and rapidly pass out of the body. So we need a regular intake throughout the day. Also, since the brain uses a very large amount of these nutrients, a short-term deficiency will affect mental abilities. While the deficiency symptoms of B vitamins are well known we still do not know exactly why many of the symptoms occur [1]. Each B vitamin has so many functions in the brain and nervous system that there are many logical explanations, but few hard proofs. Many people choose to safeguard against deficiency by taking a B complex supplement every day.

Niacin and Pantothenic Acid

Of all the nutrients connected with mental health niacin, (vitamin B3), is the most famous. Niacin was first discovered because deficiency was identified as the cause of 'pellagra', a disease in which people developed mental illness, diarrhoea and eczema. Due to the pioneering work of Drs Abram Hoffer and Humphrey Osmond, niacin has been extensively researched as a treatment for schizophrenia and found highly effective in acute schizophrenia in doses of several grams (see Chapter 16). The RDA is only 18mg!

Getting enough niacin does more than stop you going crazy. In one study, 141mg of niacin every day improved memory by 10 to 40% in both young and old people [2].

Pantothenic acid, also called vitamin B5, is another potent memory booster. It is needed to make both stress hormones, and also the vital memory-coding neurotransmitter, acetylcholine. Supplementing extra, particularly with choline, may improve your memory (see Chapter 10).

Vitamins B6, B12 and Folic Acid

It is very important for pregnant women to get enough B6 because it is essential for the proper development of the central nervous system and brain. A lack of B6 interferes with the brain's receptors for glutamate-based neurotransmitters which are involved in learning and memory [3].

B6 is also needed to form serotonin, another key brain chemical. In one study, the level of psychological distress in HIV infected people decreased as their B6 status improved through supplementation [4]. Adding tryptophan further reduced the level of distress. So B6 protects you from stress.

Folic acid is often deficient in mental health patients. So much so that consultant psychiatrist, Dr Carney from Lancaster Moor Hospital recommends that folate deficiency is common enough in the mentally ill to justify carrying out serum folate and B12 estimations as a routine admission procedure [5]. Like B6, getting enough in pregnancy is vital,

NUTRIENT	EFFECTS OF DEFICIENCY	FOOD SOURCES
B3	Depression, psychosis	Wholegrains, vegetables
B6	Irritability, poor memory	Wholegrains, bananas
FOLIC ACID	Anxiety, depression	Green leafy vegetables
B12	Confusion, poor memory	Cheese, eggs
ZINC	Confusion, blank mind, apathy	Oysters, nuts, seeds, fish
MAGNESIUM	Irritability, insomnia, depression	Vegetables, nuts, seeds
MANGANESE	Dizziness, convulsions	Nuts, seeds, tropical fruit
ESSENTIAL FATS	Depression, mood swings, Poor memory, learning difficulties	Nuts, seeds and oils

both for protecting against spina bifida and also for general intellectual development. While folic acid deficiency is associated with depression, dementia and poor mental function in the elderly, children born to folic acid deficient mothers show delayed intellectual development [6]. Supplementing folic acid can help a significant proportion of people suffering from mental illness (although not if they're histadelic - see Chapter 14). In a recent study at the Department of Psychiatry at King's College Hospital in London, a third of 123 patients were found to have low levels of folic acid. They were then given either folic acid or placebos for six months. There was a significant improvement only in the group of patients taking folic acid, which included both depressed and schizophrenic patients [7].

Vitamin B12 is also vital for a healthy nervous system. Without it neither the senses, nor the brain work properly. Deficiency has been shown to be present in as much as half of patients with dementia, with an equivalent number showing an inability to absorb it [8]. Taking extra B12 does reverse brain and sensory abnormalities, although it doesn't cure dementia.

Vitamins B6, B12 and folic acid have something in common. They are needed to control the use of sulfur-containing amino acids. Without them unwanted by-products of metabolism, such as homocysteine, can build up and over-stimulate the brain, producing anxiety and mental illness. They each have so many critical roles to play in the brain and nervous system that ensuring you are getting optimal levels of these nutrients is a prerequisite for mental health.

Vitamin C

Vitamin C does more than stop you getting colds. It has many roles to play in the brain, helping to balance neurotransmitters. While not so spectacular as niacin, vitamin C has been shown to reduce the symptoms of schizophrenia [9]. A number of studies have shown that people diagnosed with mental illness may have much greater requirements of this vitamin, and are frequently deficient [10]. In one study patients only started to excrete the same amount of vitamin C as the control group when given 1 gram a day, ten times the RDA. Dr Vandercamp, from the VA Hospital in Michigan, found that schizophrenic patients could metabolise ten times more vitamin C than normal people 11. Vitamin C deficiency is also far more common than realised in mentally ill people, often because they don't look after themselves properly and eat poorly. Pronounced vitamin C deficiency can make you crazy, as reported by Professor Derri Shtasel from the department of psychiatry at the University of Pennsylvania School of Medicine in Philadelphia. She describes a case of a woman who presented with confusion and hearing voices, plus physical symptoms. She was tested for vitamin C status and found to be very deficient. After being given vitamin C she had fewer hallucinations, her speech improved and she became more motivated and sociable 12.

Calcium & Magnesium - Natural Tranquillisers

'My nerves are shot to pieces'. That's how many of us instinctively describe our state when we're feeling anxious, edgy and unable to relax. Our nerves send messages through a series of chemicals, which change the positive or negative charge of our nerve cells. This difference in charge creates a current of electricity passing on the nervous signal. Just like an out of tune car, these signals can become out of tune. Calcium collects inside and outside the cell, to help turn on a signal. When there is too much intracellular calcium (which can be caused by not enough dietary calcium) a state of tension predominates. Cramps are an obvious example of this. On the other hand, magnesium acts to relax the cell signal, and therefore a lack of magnesium helps create that edgy feeling.

"A lack of magnesium increases one's nervousness, irritability and aggression", says Dr Krehl. The British Medical Journal reports that magnesium deficiency can induce B1 deficiency, bringing on apathy and depression. Two American psychiatrists discovered that a build up of lactic acid brought on symptoms of impending doom, fear of insanity, fear of heart attacks and difficulty breathing. When calcium was administered the fears diminished. These results were confirmed in a controlled experiment, and it is thought that calcium binds to lactic acid, forming calcium lactate, which is quite harmless. Magnesium has also been used successfully to treat autistic children, together with other nutrients.

Next time you reach for a sleeping pill reach for calcium and magnesium instead. As a natural sleeping aid 600mg of calcium and

400mg of magnesium usually does the trick.

Magnesium has many roles to play in the nervous system and the possibility of magnesium deficiency being a cause of mental illness is starting to be researched more thoroughly. When patients are put on psychotropic drugs both calcium and magnesium levels tend to decline[13]. Supplementing them helps to reduce unpleasant side-effects.

Magnesium is perhaps the second most commonly deficient mineral. Without it it's easy to become 'wound up', anxious, hyperactive and irritable. Other symptoms to watch out for as possible signs of magnesium deficiency are muscle cramps, tremors or spasms, high blood pressure, irregular heartbeat, constipation and fits or convulsions.

Magnesium is rich in green, leafy vegetables because it is part of the chlorophyll molecule, which makes plants green. It's also rich in nuts and seeds, particularly sesame, sunflower and pumpkin seeds. An ideal intake is probably 500mg a day, which is almost double what most people achieve. A tablespoon of seeds a day, plus 200mg in a multimineral, is a good way to ensure you're getting enough.

Manganese - The Forgotten Mineral

Too much and too little manganese affects the way our brain functions. An excess, found occasionally in miners inhaling dust from manganese ore, results in psychosis and nervous disorders similar to Parkinson's disease. However, excess is rare.

Too little manganese may also be a contributive factor for schizophrenia and other psychotic problems. Even as early as 1917 manganese chloride was found to be effective for the treatment of schizophrenia. Dr Carl Pfeiffer revived the interest in these trace metals, and has found that almost all patients can benefit from extra manganese and zinc [14]. He found that high levels of copper or iron displace manganese and help to produce the continuous and excessive over stimulation that characterises so many psychotic states. He also found that slight manganese deficiency is associated with insomnia, restlessness, non-productive activity and elevated blood pressure. Clearly one doesn't have to be psychotic to experience these common signs of deficiency.

Epilepsy may also be associated with deficiency of manganese although the mechanism is not completely understood. Sohler in 1979, clearly showed that epileptics have significantly lower manganese levels than other people 15. Drugs used to treat some forms of mental illness can produce the unfortunate side effects of an involuntary twitching of the facial muscles. Since the drugs, called phenothiazines, have been found to attach to manganese, making it less available for use in the brain, one researcher hypothesised that manganese might be useful for preventing the side effects caused by these anti-psychotic drugs. Out of fifteen people given manganese supplementation, seven were cured outright of their involuntary muscle twitches, three were much improved, and four were improved. Only one person did not respond.

Why Your Diet May Be Manganese Deficient

Like many trace minerals, the difference between the amount required to prevent deficiency and the levels of manganese for optimum health vary considerably. While the US National Research Council recommends between 2.5 and 5 mg a day for a 70 kg man, some people have been known to only respond when given 300 mg a day! 16 Most researchers agree that the requirement for manganese ranges between 2 and 20 mg a day. The average person in Britain gets 4.6 mg from diet (up to 50 % of which is from drinking tea), leaving those with a greater need for manganese, deficient. Since the mineral is found mainly in seeds, nuts and grains, junk food diets high in refined foods are most likely to be deficient. Manganese-rich foods are leafy green vegetables, beets, pineapple, bran, wheat, egg yolk, kelp, nuts, seeds and tropical fruit.

Manganese is also extremely poorly absorbed and easily excreted from the body. In cows, as little as one per cent is taken from their diet. Manganese appears to be absorbed through the same pathway as iron, and an excess of iron can interfere with absorption. For these reasons manganese supplementation can often help to ensure that adequate levels are obtained. Since excess manganese is readily excreted there is no danger of taking too much. Most manganese supplements contain between 5 and 25mg of this mineral.

Zinc - The Mental Element

Zinc is perhaps the most commonly deficient mineral, and the most critical nutrient for mental health. The average intake in Britain is 7.5mg, which is half the RDA of 15mg. This means that half the British population get less than half the level of zinc thought to protect against deficiency. Zinc deficiency is associated with schizophrenia, depression, anxiety, anorexia, delinquency, hyperactivity, autism - in short, almost all types of mental health problems. For this reason there is a whole chapter (Chapter 17) which explores the connections.

There are also many circumstances that increase one's need for zinc, quite apart from not getting enough from diet. These include stress, infections, PMS and other hormone imbalances, using the contraceptive pill, excess copper, frequent alcohol consumption, blood sugar problems and an inherited extra need for zinc. It is very easy to become severely deficient through a collection of circumstances, as the case of David illustrates.

David was diagnosed as suffering from schizophrenia at the age of 20, having suffered from acute depression, paranoia and extreme mental confusion. He was also hearing and seeing things. His doctor prescribed the drug Stelazine to calm him down, but the drug (as with other similar drugs) just cut the edge off all feelings. He still couldn't go back to college or relate with his friends and family in a normal way.

Symptoms of mental illness can, and often are, the result of an inborn genetic tendency to biochemical imbalances, coupled with poor nutrition from the outside. With a history of meningitis, hyperactivity, eczema and asthma as a child and mild gout in his teenage years, I suspected a genetic factor, possibly revolving around zinc and the immune system which are associated with all these problems.

Before his 'schizophrenic' breakdown, David had been globe trotting. He'd been to Morocco and India, drinking and smoking considerable amounts of alcohol and cannabis. Both these drugs deplete zinc stores and are potent immune suppressors. His diet, which was not very good and mainly vegetarian, would not have provided enough zinc and other nutrients. He contracted jaundice in Morocco and amoebic dysentery in India, plus a severe bout of 'flu'. These infections knock the immune system for six and deplete zinc stores even further. Tests revealed chronic B6 and zinc deficiency. The symptoms often include low energy, confusion, 'blank' mind, poor skin, pallor, frequent infections, white marks on the nails and an inability to deal with stress.

Within days of adding B6 and zinc supplements plus a diet rich in fruit and vegetables, and avoiding sugar, coffee and alcohol, he became symptom free. I wrote to his doctor requesting he stop Stelazine, which he did. He still remained free from all his symptoms and looked and felt much healthier. Some months later he got a place at a top college to continue his studies. Last time I spoke to him, two years later, he hadn't had any return of his previous symptoms. This year he is due to qualify with a degree.

4

FATS FOR THE BRAIN

F at is good for you. In fact, it is totally essential for optimal health. Essential fats reduce the risk for cancer, heart disease, allergies, arthritis, eczema, infections, as well as depression, fatigue, schizophrenia, PMS and promote maximum mental performance [1]. Twenty per cent of the dry weight of the brain is made up of essential fats [2].

If you are fat-phobic you are depriving yourself of essential health-giving nutrients. The same is true if the fat you eat is hard fat - from dairy products, margarines or meat. In fact, unless you go out of your way to eat the right kind of fat-rich foods, or supplement essential oils the chances are you're malnourished. Most people in Britain are overnourished in saturated fats, the fats that kill, and undernourished in essential fats, the fats that heal.

Fat Figures

To put this into figures it is considered optimum to consume no more than 20% of overall calories as fat. The current average in Britain is above 40%. Countries who have a low incidence of fat-related diseases like Japan, Thailand and the Phillipines, consume only about 15% of total calorie intake as fat. For example, Japanese people eat 40 grams of fat a day. British people eat 142 grams of fat a day.

Most authorities now agree that, of our total fat intake, no more than one-third should be saturated (hard) fat, and at least one third should be polyunsaturated oils providing the two essential fats: the linoleic acid family, known as Omega 6; and the alpha-linolenic acid family, known as Omega 3. (More on these in a minute.) These two essential fat families also need to be in balance. The ideal balance is probably close to twice as much Omega 6 as Omega 3. So an ideal 'fat profile' might be 5% Omega 6 + 2.5% Omega 3 + 7.5% mono-unsaturated fat + 7.5% saturated fat = 20%.

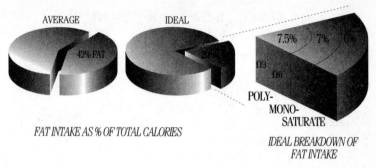

FAT INTAKE AS % OF TOTAL CALORIES

IDEAL BREAKDOWN OF
FAT INTAKE

Figure 3 - Average vs Ideal Fat Intake

Most people are deficient in both Omega 6 and Omega 3 fats. In addition, a high intake of saturated fats and damaged polyunsaturated fats, known as 'trans' fats, stops the body making good use of the little essential fats the average person eats in a day.

The 'Omega 6' Fat Family

The grandmother of the Omega 6 fat family is linoleic acid. Linoleic acid is converted by the body into gamma-linolenic acid (GLA), provided you've got enough vitamin B6, biotin, zinc and magnesium to drive the enzyme that makes the conversion. Evening primrose oil and borage oil are the richest known sources of GLA and, by supplementing these direct, you need take in less overall oil to get an optimal intake of Omega 6 fats. The ideal intake is probably around 150mg of GLA a day, which is equivalent to 1,500mg of evening primrose oil, or 750mg of high-potency borage oil - a capsule a day.

GLA then gets converted into DGLA and from there into 'prostaglandins' which are extremely active hormone-like substances in the body. The particular kind of prostaglandins made from these Omega 6 oils are called 'Series 1 prostaglandins'. These keep the blood thin, relax blood vessels therefore lowering blood pressure, help to maintain water balance in the body, boost immunity, decrease inflammation and pain and help insulin to work which is good for blood sugar balance. This is the short-list. As every year passes more and more health-promoting functions are being found. Prostaglandins themselves cannot be supplemented as they are very short-lived.

Omega 6 Deficiency Signs

Do you have high blood pressure?
Do you suffer from PMS or breast pain?
Do you suffer from eczema or dry skin?
Do you suffer from dry eyes?
Do you have an inflammatory health problem?
Do you have chronic fatigue?
Do you have a blood sugar problem or diabetes?
Do you have multiple sclerosis?
Do you drink alcohol every day?
Do you have depression or mood swings?
Do you suffer from excessive thirst?

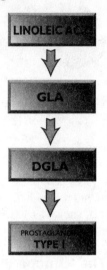

Five or more 'yes' answers indicates that you may be deficient in Omega 6 fats. Check your diet carefully for the foods listed below.

Instead we rely on a good intake of Omega 6 fats from which the body can make the prostaglandins we need.

The Memory Booster

Omega 6 fats are also essential for mental health. Of all the tissues of the body, the brain has the highest proportion of Omega 6 fats. They are part of the nerve tissue and influence brain function. Numerous studies have shown that schizophrenics have low levels [3]. A survey by the World Health Organisation found that the countries which had the most severe schizophrenia had the lowest intake of essential fats.

Trials with Omega 6 fats such as evening primrose oil have had mixed results. However, a more recent large-scale placebo controlled trial using evening primrose oil showed significant improvement [4]. However, results became even more spectacular when vitamins B6, zinc, niacin and vitamin C were added, all of which are needed by the body to turn essential fats into prostaglandins. This produced marked improvements in memory, schizophrenia symptoms and also tardive dyskinesia, a side-effect of medication.

Adding evening primrose oil to the diet of alcoholics going through withdrawal dramatically reduces symptoms and, in the long-term, improves memory 5. Due to its reported effects on memory evening primrose oil was given to Alzheimers patients in a controlled trial. Once again, highly significant improvements in memory were found 6.

This family of fats comes exclusively from seeds and their oils. The best seed oils are hemp, pumpkin, sunflower, safflower, sesame, corn, walnut, soybean and wheatgerm oil. About half the fat in these oils comes from the Omega 6 family, mainly as linoleic acid. An optimal intake is 1 to 2 tablespoons a day, or 2 to 3 tablespoons of ground seeds.

The 'Omega 3' Fat Family

The modern day diet is likely to be more deficient in Omega 3 fats than Omega 6 fats simply because the grandmother of the Omega 3 family, alpha-linolenic acid, and her metabolically active grandchildren, EPA (Eicosapentaenoic acid) and DHA (docosahexaenoic acid), from which Prostaglandin Series 3 are made, are more unsaturated and more prone to damage in cooking and food processing. In fact, the average person today gets one sixth of the Omega 3 fats found in the diet of those in 1850, partly due to food choices, but mainly due to food processing.

As these fats get converted in the body to more 'active' substances they become more unsaturated and, generally the word used for them gets longer (e.g. oleic acid - one degree of unsaturation; linoleic - 2 degrees of unsaturation; linolenic - 3 degrees of unsaturation; Eicosapentaenoic - 5 degrees of unsaturation etc.). You can see this increasing complexity as we move up the food chain. For example, plankton, the staple food of small fish, is rich in alpha-linolenic acid. Carnivorous fish, like mackerel or herring, eat the small fish who have converted some of their alpha-linolenic acid to more complex fats. The carnivorous fish continue the conversion. Seals eat them and have the highest EPA and DHA concentration, then Eskimos eat the seals and benefit from the ready-made meal of EPA and DHA from which they can easily make the series 3 prostaglandins.

Increased Learning Potential

These prostaglandins are also essential for proper brain function, affecting vision, learning ability, co-ordination and mood, reduce the

Omega 3 Deficiency Signs

Do you have dry skin?

Do you have any inflammatory health problems?

Do you suffer from water retention?

Do you get tingling in the arms or legs?

Do you have high blood pressure or high triglycerides?

Are you prone to infections?

Are you finding it harder to lose weight?

Has your memory and learning ability declined?

Do you suffer from a lack of co-ordination or impaired vision?

LINOLENIC ACID

↓

EPA

PROSTAGLANDIN TYPE 3   DHA

If a child, are you small for your age or growing slowly?

Five or more 'yes' answers indicates that you may be deficient in Omega 3 fats. Check your diet carefully for the foods listed below.

stickiness of blood, as well as controlling blood cholesterol and fat levels, improving immune function, metabolism, reducing inflammation and maintaining water balance.

In fact, the level of the Omega 3 fats, DHA and EPA, are markers for intelligence. Studies have found that the blood levels of these essential fats correlates with intellectual performance and learning ability at the age of 5 [7]. The World Health organisation now recommend that formula feeds include these oils which, when added, increase the blood levels of these vital nerve nutrients [8].

An on-going research programme at Hammersmith Hospital has identified that the babies of vegan breast-feeding mothers are brainier, probably because their breast milk, compared to the milk of dairy-eating vegetarians or omnivores or bottle milk, provides more of the essential fatty acids needed for the development of neural membranes.

According to Louise Thomas, a member of the Hammersmith team, the balance of saturated vs polyunsaturated fat in fat tissue could act as a marker for intelligence [9].

Donald Rudin, a doctor and medical researcher, has shown that flax oil, rich in Omega 3, can improve the behaviour of schizophrenics and juvenile delinquents who fail to respond to counselling [10]. It can also improve visual function, colour perception and mental acuity.

The best seed oils for Omega 3 fats are flax (also known as linseed), hemp and pumpkin. In much the same way as evening primrose oil bypasses the first 'conversion' stage of linoleic acid, eating carnivorous fish or their oils bypasses the first two conversion stages of alpha-linolenic acid, to provide EPA and DHA. This is why fish eaters like the Japanese have three times the Omega 3 fats in their body fat than the average American. Vegans, who eat more seeds and nuts, have twice the Omega 3 fat level in their body fat than the average American.

Essential Balance

While borage oil or evening primrose oil may be the best source of Omega 6 and fish oil the best source of Omega 3, that doesn't make them the best allrounder. The ideal source of essential fats should have high levels of both. Differing views exist about the ideal ratio. Estimated intakes of our hunter-gatherer ancestors suggest that we need equal amounts. The ratio found in blood even of high fish eaters is about 5 times as much Omega 6, suggesting that it is either relatively more important, or that all cultures have a relatively greater deficiency of Omega 3 fats. Some researchers advise that we may need to take in twice as much Omega 6 as Omega 3 to match our relative need. Either of these ratios is along way off the average diet, which is deficient in both, however with at least ten times more Omega 6 than Omega 3 fat.

The best in this respect is hemp seed oil from the marijuana plant. Hemp has been grown for many years. The fibre is used to make rope, the seeds can be used to make hemp butter and the leaves are a good fertiliser. It is, however, illegal to grow in many parts of the world. The seeds and fibre are legal, neither of which will make you high, and can therefore be imported into the UK. Hemp is now making a comeback, both as a source of nutrition, and as a fabric for clothes. Hemp seed oil is 19% alpha-linolenic acid (Omega 3), 57% linoleic acid and 2% GLA (both Omega 6). It is the only common seed oil that meets all known essential fatty acid needs.

Another way of meeting the needs for both Omega 3 and Omega 6 fats is to combine seeds. Sunflower and sesame are good sources of Omega 3, pumpkin provides reasonable quantities of both, and flax seed is richest in Omega 3, being approximately 50% Omega 3 and 10% Omega 6. Put 1 measure each of sesame, sunflower and pumpkin seeds and 2 measures of flax seeds in a sealed jar and keep it in the fridge, away from light, heat and oxygen. Simply adding 2 tablespoons of these seeds ground to your breakfast each morning guarantees a good daily intake of essential fatty acids. Alternatively, add 1 and make up the difference with a salad dressing, nuts or seeds later in the day.

Of these seeds the most unsaturated is flax seed and hence it is the most prone to damage. For this reason its important to buy fresh seeds that have been properly stored minimising heat, light and oxygen exposure. Some companies offer seed oils that are processed in such a way as to protect the oils from oxidation, thus preserving their essential fat status. We recommend you only buy oils that are extracted from organic seeds, cold-pressed to minimise heat, and stored in a light-proof container. In this case a good daily balance of essential fatty acids could be obtained by 1 tablespoon of flax seed oil or a high potency capsule of EPA/DHA **plus** 2 tablespoons of ground seeds (e.g sesame, sunflower and pumpkin) or a high potency evening primrose oil or borage oil capsule.

Each of the following provides approximately your daily need for these essential fatty acids. Individual needs do, however, vary so this is only a rough guideline.

OMEGA 3	OMEGA 6
2.5% to 5% of total calories	5% of total calories
8 to 17grams a day	17grams a day
Hemp seed oil 1 tablespoon	Hemp seed oil 1 tablespoon
Flax seed Oil 1 tablespoon	Evening primrose oil 1,000mg
Flax seeds 2 tablespoons	Borage oil 500mg
EPA/DHA 1,000mg	Sunflower seeds 1 tablespoon
Pumpkin seeds 4 tablespoons	Pumpkin seeds 2 tablespoons
	Sesame seeds 1.5 tablespoons

5

BRAIN POLLUTION

Optimum brain nutrition isn't just about getting the right nutrients. Since our bodies, brains and nervous systems are literally made from what we take in – through food, air and water – there is every reason to consider that changes in diet, pollution and environment could have a bearing on physical and mental health. The effects of recreational drugs like alcohol, or prescription drugs like anti–depressants, illustrate the powerful influence of chemicals on mood and behaviour.

In the last 50 years alone, 3,500 new chemicals have been added to food. A further 3,000 have been introduced into our homes [1]. Heavy metals like lead and cadmium are so commonplace in a 20th century environment that the average person has 700 times higher body levels than our ancestors [2]. Most of our food is sprayed with pesticides and herbicides such that the average person may have up to a gallon sprayed on the fruit and vegetables they consume in a year [3].

All of these are classified as anti–nutrients – substances that interfere either with our ability to absorb or to use essential nutrients, and in some cases, promote the loss of essential nutrients from the body.

Nobody really knows to what extent this modern cocktail of anti–nutrients messes up our mental health, however we do know that high intakes of lead, cadmium, certain food colourings and other chemicals can have a disastrous effect on intellectual performance and behaviour.

A high intake of anti–nutrients has been associated with mood swings, poor impulse control and aggressive behaviour, poor attention span, depression and apathy, disturbed sleep patterns, impaired memory and intellectual performance. If these kind of symptoms are present, the nutritional approach to promoting mental health includes testing for high levels of anti–nutrients and, if found, removing the source and detoxifying the body. Here are some examples of

ANTI–NUTRIENT	EFFECT	SOURCE	ANTAGONIST
Lead	Hyperactivity, aggression	Exhaust fumes	Vitamin C, Zinc
Cadmium	Aggression, confusion	Cigarettes	Vitamin C, Zinc
Mercury	Headaches, memory loss	Pesticides, fillings	Selenium
Aluminium	Associated with senility	Cookware, water	Zinc, Magnesium
Copper	Anxiety & phobia	Water	Zinc
Tartrazine	Hyperactivity	Food colourings	Zinc

anti–nutrients, their source, effects in excess on mental health, and nutritional antagonists which help to lower body levels of these unwanted substances.

Heavy Metal Kids

Researchers at the California Institute of Technology have been studying changes in lead concentrations throughout the world - in ocean beds, soil samples and even snow. Their work shows that lead concentration, even in unpolluted Greenland, has risen between 500 and 1,000 times since prehistoric ages. Most of this increase has taken place in the past 100 years, and is mainly a result of industrial lead pollution and lead exhaust from cars. Comparisons of lead found in humans showed a similar 500 to 1,000 fold increase. How can we be sure that we are designed to eliminate such large levels of lead? We cannot.

Of course, the question we must first ask is: at what level does lead have any adverse effect? The guidelines from different countries vary quite considerably. In Britain the blood levels allowed in industrial workers are 80mcg/dl (micrograms per decilitre) for men and 40kmcg/dl for women. In the USA the level is 40mcg/dl regardless of sex. The much criticised DHSS 'Lawther Report', published in 1980, recommended 35mcg/dl as the safe level for lead measured in blood.

Yet three recent research studies have all shown conclusively that levels of lead as low as 13mcg/dl can affect behaviour and lower intelligence in children. When we consider that the average EEC lead level in the 1980's was 13mcg/dl we must come to the appalling conclusion that lead was then damaging the minds of one in two children in the EEC. With more and more people switching to lead-free petrol the situation is improving.

The Needleman Study

The first study to shake the status quo on lead toxicity was the Needleman study. Herbert Needleman, Associate Professor of child psychiatry, looked at a group of 2,146 children in first and second grade schools in Birmingham, USA. He examined lead concentrations in shed baby teeth to obtain more long term levels than shown by a simple blood test. He then asked the school teachers to rate the behaviour of children they had taught for at least two months. This was done using a questionnaire designed to measure the teacher's rating of children for a number of characteristics. He also ran a series of behavioural, intellectual and physiological tests on each child before dividing the children into six groups according to their lead concentration in teeth.

His results showed a clear relationship between lead concentrations and bad school behaviour, as rated by the teachers without any knowledge of the children's lead levels. Needleman also found the average IQ for the high lead children was 4.5 points below that of the low lead group. Reaction time (a measure of attention capability) was also consistently worse in those with higher lead levels. Even EEG readings (which measure brain wave patterns) showed clear differences, based on lead concentration. Perhaps the most interesting result was that none of the high lead children had an IQ above 125 points (100 is average), compared to 5% in the low lead group.

Needleman's study shows that although the behaviour and intelligence of normal children are clearly affected by lead, we cannot be sure of the severity of the problem in Britain. Nor can we determine safe blood levels for lead concentration, since his study used teeth. The use of teeth identified the need for more long-term measures, but is not the most practical for screening purposes! A DHSS screening programme based on yanking your teeth out could hardly be considered progress. For these reasons we must next consider the work of Richard Lansdown.

The Lansdown Study

Richard Lansdown, principal psychologist at the London Hospital for Sick Children, and William Yule, psychologist at the University of London, decided to replicate the essentials of Needleman's study on London children using blood lead levels instead of teeth. The children selected had an average blood lead level of 13.52mcg/dl (35mcg/dl is the 'safe' level recommended by the Lawther Report in 1980). This is similar to other national studies of mean lead levels. Again the children's behaviour was rated by the teachers, and IQ and other tests were made. Lansdown's results were even more striking than Needleman's. The difference in IQ score between high and low lead children was seven IQ points - even though none of the children had lead levels above 35mcg'dl, the 'safe' DHSS level. In fact, the 'threshold' level for safety based on this study would be 12mcg/dl. Once again, none of the high lead group children had IQ's above 125, while in the low lead group, 5% did.

The Winneke Study

A further study of Gerhard Winneke PhD, Director of the Medical Institute of Environmental Hygiene in Dusseldorf, found essentially the same results. He studied 458 children with an average blood level of 14.2mcg/dl, and found an IQ deficit of five to seven points between those with high and low lead levels. Winneke also looked at dentine (teeth) levels and found a close correlation to blood - a further confirmation for Needleman's results.

Are You at Risk?

Although adults are not safe from lead poisoning, it is children who are most at risk. This is especially so up to age 12, when lead can create irreversible brain damage. Children also absorb lead more easily and are frequently exposed to higher concentrations in dust.

This means that a proportion of children, particularly in cities, are absorbing enough lead to affect their intellectual development. The most common symptoms in children are an inability to concentrate, disturbed sleep patterns, uncharacteristic aggressive outbursts, fussiness about food, sinus conditions and headaches. Children from birth to age eight are most at risk, with a peak around age two to three, although it is only the size of the problem that diminishes from age eight - the problem doesn't disappear. Adults are more likely to experience a chronic lack of physical and mental energy, together with headaches, depression and loss of memory.

An EEC survey of lead levels in Britain in 1980 showed that levels were higher in inner cities than outer cities, with an average inner city level of 12.8 mcg/dl. London was the least polluted city, Leeds and Manchester were the most. Men had higher lead levels, as did smokers and people living in pre-1940 housing, presumably due to the use of lead pipes. However, rural areas did not register dramatically lower lead levels. Fortunately, these levels are now falling.

Cadmium is another heavy metal that is associated with disturbed mental performance and increased aggression. The most common source is in cigarettes. Cadmium levels in the blood correlate well to the number of cigarettes smoked. There is also cadmium in car exhaust fumes and in food, especially if it's refined since beneficial minerals which act as cadmium antagonists are no longer present.

Aluminium is in widespread use in food packaging and will turn up in many common household products. It's in antacids, toothpaste tubes, aluminium foil, pots and pans and water. There is an association between aluminium and Alzheimers, discussed in Chapter 25. Not all aluminium will enter the body. Only under certain circumstances will aluminium leach, for example, from a pan. Old fashioned aluminium cookware, if used to boil something acidic like tea or rhubarb, will leach particles of aluminium into the water. The more zinc deficient you are the more you absorb.

Mercury is the reason why hatters went mad. By polishing top hats with mercury they became overloaded with this toxic element which disturbs brain function and makes you crazy. Mercury is very toxic indeed and small amounts reach us from contaminated foods. Of particular concern is fish caught in polluted waters. Mercury is used in a number of chemical processes and accidents and illegal dumping has led to increased mercury levels in some areas, including the Channel. Fish, especially larger fish like tuna, store the mercury which we then ingest. Fortunately, tuna is also high in selenium, a mercury antagonist.

Analyses of thousands of hair, blood and sweat samples of people in Britain by Dr Stephen Davies, of the Biolab Medical Unit in London, has clearly shown that each of these toxic elements accumulates with age [4]. Simultaneously, levels of essential elements decline, leading him to conclude that our overexposure to toxic elements and underconsumption of essential elements has exceeded the human body's capacity to adapt and successfully detoxify. The lack of sufficient essential elements makes lead, cadmium, mercury and aluminium even more toxic [5]. The combination of these factors is no doubt lowering our overall intellectual performance and emotional stability.

Detoxifying Brain Pollutants

Once we've ingested toxic metals they must compete with other minerals for absorption. These minerals are called antagonists and form our first line of defence. Once the element has been absorbed, some natural body substances latch on to it and try to take it out of the body. These are called chelators (pronounced key-lay-tors). It is the latter principle which lies behind the administration of two drugs, penicillamine and EDTA.

Vitamin C Lowers Lead Levels

One of the problems with lead poisoning is that once it is in the brain, where most damage is done, it is very difficult to remove it. Neither penicillamine nor the more potent EDTA chelating drugs have much effect, because neither can readily cross the blood-brain barrier. But vitamin C can. In a study on rats with a lead concentration of 1.7 in the brain, administering EDTA resulted in a drop to 1.56. But vitamin C caused a drop to 1.33.

Another substance known to lower lead is zinc which acts as an antagonist to lead by preventing its absorption in the gut. One study by Dr Carl Pfeiffer administered 2,000mg of vitamin C and 60mg of zinc (as zinc gluconate) to 22 workers at a lead battery plant, all of whom had elevated lead levels. Complete blood tests were taken at the start of the study and after 6, 12 and 24 weeks. The average blood lead level at the start was 62.1mcg/dl. The workers were still receiving similar exposure at work even though there was a steady decrease of lead levels over the 24 week period. Nineteen out of 22 had a decline in blood lead levels, and those with the highest initial lead experienced the greatest change in lead levels. One dropped 35mcg/dl, while six dropped more than 20mcg/dl and nine dropped more than 10mcg/dl. Calcium is effective at keeping down lead levels, since lead otherwise stores more easily in our bones. Keeping calcium levels topped up pushes out this environmental poison. Calcium is also particularly effective at keeping down cadmium and aluminium levels.

Vitamin C is an all rounder too. It has the ability to latch on to heavy metals in the blood and escort them out, sacrificing itself in the process. So high metal burdens call for more vitamin C. It is effective for removing lead, arsenic and cadmium and is a most important part of any detoxification programme. Phosphorus is another mineral which can help prevent the ravages of lead. At a conference on lead and health, Professor Bryce-Smith said: 'Dietary manipulation and the provision of a calcium and phosphate supplement may both be helpful'.

Zinc Counteracts Cadmium

Zinc was the partner used in the Pfeiffer study, and has been shown to be good at reducing body levels of lead and cadmium. A previous study by the Princeton Bio Center achieved a 25% drop in lead levels. These results show clearly that there is no need to use toxic chelators when nutritional ones can do the job perfectly well. Indeed, most of us could benefit from extra zinc. Pectin is derived from apples. Bananas, carrots and citrus fruits are also excellent sources. These chelate heavy metals in the same way as alginic acid in seaweeds, promoting your health. One more reason for an apple a day.

Selenium Protects Against Mercury

Selenium is a mercury antagonist, and protects us from the mercury present in most seafood. Supplementing an extra dose is always a good idea if there are signs of excess mercury. It also has a similar relationship with arsenic and cadmium, although it is not so pronounced.

Sulphur-containing amino acids are found as the proteins in garlic, onions and eggs. The specific amino acids are called methionine and cystine and protect against mercury, cadmium and lead toxicity.

Food Additives Questioned

Tartrazine is one of many chemical additives known to provoke allergic reactions that affect mental health. Over 200,000 tonnes of chemical additives are added to food each year, or approximately 10lbs per person. Some of us, perhaps all of us, aren't coping well with this level of chemical onslaught.

Dr Neil Ward, from the University of Surrey, found that adding tartrazine to drinks increased the amount of zinc excreted in the urine, perhaps by binding to zinc in the blood and preventing it from being used by the body[6]. In this study they also found emotional and behavioural changes in every child who drank the drink containing tartrazine. Four out of the ten children in the study had severe reactions, three developing eczema or asthma within 45 minutes of ingestion. At this point in time we really have no idea what the combined effect of the literally thousands of man-made chemicals have on health.

A nutrition counsellor can test for the presence of many of these anti–nutrients and devise a lifestyle, diet and supplement programme to eliminate this potential contributor to mental instability. The consequence of decreasing the burden of these anti-nutrients is a greater ability to cope with the unavoidable stresses life gives us to deal with and improve mental performance.

6

BEATING THE SUGAR BLUES

The most important nutrient of all for the brain and nervous system is its fuel - glucose. Any imbalance in the supply of glucose to the brain and you can experience fatigue, irritability, dizziness, insomnia, excessive sweating especially at night, poor concentration and forgetfulness, excessive thirst, depression and crying spells, digestive disturbances and blurred vision. Research at the Massachusetts Institute of Technology found a massive 26% difference between the IQ scores of children whose consumption of refined carbohydrates was in the top fifth of the population, compared to those who were in the bottom fifth. To maximise mental performance you need an even supply of glucose to the brain, to maintain a good level of mental energy.

What you experience as energy, whether mental or physical, is the end result of a series of chemical reactions that takes place in every cell in your body. The process that turns food into energy is called catabolism. By a carefully controlled sequence of chemical reactions, food is broken down into its component parts, and these are combusted with oxygen, to make a unit of cellular energy called ATP, which in turn makes muscles work, nerve signals fire and brain cells function. Light years ahead of man's primitive attempts to produce energy, this magical process happens inside every single cell and the only waste products are water and carbon dioxide. But first of all, the fuel has to be refined.

Food for Fuel

Although we can make energy from protein, fat and carbohydrate, carbohydrate rich foods are the best kind of fuel. This is because when fat and protein are used to make energy there is a build up of toxic

43

substances in the body. Carbohydrates are the only 'smokeless' fuel. Carbohydrates can be divided into starches (or complex carbohydrates) and sugars (or simple carbohydrates). Grains, lentils, beans and vegetables, especially potatoes, all contain complex carbohydrates, while fruit, all forms of sugar, including honey, and some vegetables contain simple carbohydrates.

Our cells need the simplest unit of carbohydrate, glucose, as fuel. So the first job of the body is to turn all forms of carbohydrate into glucose. This is the end goal of digestion. Special glands in the mouth, pancreas and small intestines secrete enzymes that gradually break down down large carbohydrate molecules into simple sugars. The same thing happens if you boil any food for long enough.

All carbohydrate food is broken down into simple forms of sugar. The three simplest forms are glucose, fructose and galactose. All these can be absorbed into the bloodstream. Malt sugar derived from grains is actually made out of two glucose molecules, known as maltose. Milk sugar is made out of a molecule of glucose and a molecule of galactose, called lactose. What we know of as sugar, whether white or brown, is actually a combination of fructose and glucose, known as sucrose. All these di-saccharides are quite rapidly broken down and absorbed into the bloodstream. Many fruits contain large amounts of fructose which requires no digestion at all.

If all you need is glucose you might think, as scientists did in the early part of this century, why not just eat sugar? By understanding what happens next you'll see why eating sugar can actually give you less energy.

Balancing Your Blood Sugar

Your bloodstream is your petrol tank. At all times it contains a relatively constant level of glucose. When your cells need energy, they can call upon your glucose stores. But just in case blood sugar levels drop too much, many cells, most notably muscle cells which use a lot of fuel, have their own reserve fuel, which is known as glycogen. The liver also carries a lot of glycogen. If you eat far more carbohydrates than you need, glucose and glycogen can be turned into a long-term storage form - fat. If really starved of fuel the body can break down protein in muscle tissue, for example, to use as fuel.

Consider the fate of a marathon runner who, over 26 miles, is going to burn a lot of fuel. As blood sugar levels drop, more and more glycogen, stored in muscles and in the liver, is converted to glucose. Once this runs out, the runner must break down fat or protein to make energy. This is far less efficient and the pain and extra effort required is known as 'hitting the wall'.

The first key for maximum energy is keeping your blood sugar level constant. The best foods for doing this are complex carbohydrates, because they break down gradually and release their sugar content slowly into the bloodstream. Fruit, which contains fructose, is also better than foods, like sugar, which rapidly break down to glucose and fructose. The reason for this is that fructose must first go to the liver where it is converted into glucose. This again slows down the increase in circulating glucose. So complex carbohydrates such as grains, beans, lentils, some vegetables and also fruit because of its fructose content, are slow-releasing forms of sugar.

Sugar and most sweeteners including honey, malt, maple syrup, molasses and very refined foods, like most biscuits, cakes, white bread and cereals, whose processing and over-cooking has already turned their complex carbohydrates into simple sugars, are fast-releasing. Hardly requiring any digestion, they release their sugar content so rapidly into the bloodstream that they are akin to putting racing fuel into a mini. The blood sugar level rises rapidly, often giving a noticeable boost to energy, then the body races to lower blood sugar levels to avoid flooding, and blood sugar levels plummet, often too low, causing a drop in energy one to three hours after eating. This is called low blood sugar, or hypoglycemia (hypo=low; glyc=sugar; emia=in the blood).

Glucose levels in the blood are our short-term storage of fuel. The more even this supply, the better our cells can function. They are neither starved nor flooded with fuel and can call on reserves when needed. The blood sugar balance is carefully controlled by hormones, chemical messengers released from endocrine glands. Insulin from the pancreas helps lower blood sugar levels by helping to transport glucose from the blood into the cells. The manufacture of insulin depends upon vitamin B6 and zinc. Another hormone-like substance with a similar effect is glucose tolerance factor (GTF). GTF is made in the liver. Its exact chemical structure is still a mystery even though it was first discovered in 1959. It contains vitamin B3, the mineral chromium and three amino acids.

Glucagon, another pancreatic hormone, can mobilise sugar stores in the muscles and liver if blood sugar levels get too low. An inability to produce insulin, or an inability to produce GTF results in elevated blood sugar levels in the blood. The cells become starved of glucose. This is diabetes, or hyperglycemia (high blood sugar). Treatment is essential, however nutritional therapy is often successful in reducing, and in some cases eliminating, the dependence on injected insulin and sometimes curing the disease.

Foods That Keep Blood Sugar Even

Foods that elevate blood sugar levels rapidly have a high score, the highest being glucose. Foods with a low score are better 'energy foods'. Notice how foods containing fructose, or complex carbohydrates, tend to have lower scores than refined foods.

The high scoring foods in the Glycemic Index chart have a pronounced effect, the low scoring foods are good to include in your diet for mental health. For example, toast, jam and cornflakes is fast releasing while porridge and pumpernickel bread is not. Of all the breads tested, French baguettes were the worst and oat cakes and slow-cook whole grain rye breads the best. Popular brands are Sonnenbrot and Volkenbrot, available in most supermarkets. Of the grain products white rice is bad news. The best was barley, followed by wholemeal spaghetti. The best fruits are apples and the best vegetables are anything raw. Cooked parsnips, carrots, beetroot and potato substantially raise blood sugar. Cooked yams, sweet potato and sweet corn had a milder effect on blood sugar levels. All pulses and dairy produce were low scoring. So a good diet includes lots of fresh vegetables and fresh fruit, beans, lentils, wholegrains, especially oats and brown rice.

The sugar content of your diet is best to decrease slowly. Gradually get used to less sweetness. For example, sweeten cereal with fruit. Dilute fruit juices until they're half juice, half water. Avoid foods with added sugar. Limit dried fruit. Eat fast releasing fruits like bananas with slow-releasing carbohydrates such as oats.

	HIGH (55+) Limit	LOW (0-54) Increase		HIGH (55+) Limit	LOW (0-54) Increase
Sugars			**Cereals**		
Glucose	100		Puffed rice	90	
Maltose	100		Cornflakes	80	
Lucozade	95		Weetabix	75	
Honey	87		Shredded wheat	67	
Mars Bar	68		Muesli	66	
Sucrose (sugar)	59		All-Bran		52
Fructose	20		Porridge oats		49
			Rice bran		19
Fruit			**Pulses**		
Watermelon	72		Baked beans (no sugar)		40
Raisins	64		Butter beans		36
Bananas	62		Chick peas		36
Orange juice		46	Blackeye beans		33
Grapes		44	Haricot beans		31
Oranges		40	Kidney beans		29
Apples		39	Lentils		29
Apple juice		37	Soya beans		15
Breads			**Dairy Products**		
French baguette	95		Yoghurt		36
Rice cakes	82		Whole milk		34
Brown bread	69		Skimmed milk		32
White bread	69				
Ryvita	69		**Vegetables (cooked)**		
Oat cakes		54	Parsnips	97	
Rye whole grain (pumpernickel)		49	Carrots	92	
			Instant potato	80	
Grain Products			New potato	70	
White rice	72		Beetroot	64	
Brown rice	66		Peas		51
Brown rice pasta	92		Yam		51
Pastry	59		Sweet potato		48
Digestive biscuits	59		Sweetcorn		48
White spaghetti		50			
Wholemeal spaghetti		42			
Barley		22			

Figure 5 - Glycemic Index of Foods

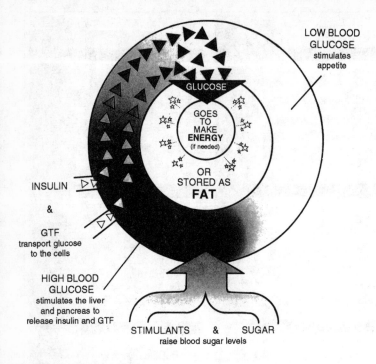

Figure 6 - The Sugar Cycle

The Sugar Blues

Frequent eating of refined sugar and carbohydrates, such as biscuits, buns, cakes and sweets, upsets this delicate balance, often resulting in glucose intolerance, an inability to maintain even blood sugar levels. The symptoms are many and include fatigue, irritability, dizziness, insomnia, excessive sweating especially at night, poor concentration and forgetfulness, excessive thirst, depression and crying spells, digestive disturbances and blurred vision.

Although they do not contain sugar as such, stimulants like coffee, tea and chocolate have much the same effect as sugar because they stimulate the liver to release stores of glucose into the blood. Once more blood sugar levels rise and so does energy. But the effect is short lived and in the long-term the regular use of such stimulants leads to lower and lower energy levels.

In the long-term, high levels of energy can only be sustained by avoiding refined carbohydrates and staying off stimulants. These substances have a double sting. While they encourage the body cells to produce energy in the short-term, they don't supply any of the vitamins, minerals or enzymes needed to turn sugar into energy. So frequent use of sugar and stimulants gradually depletes vital vitamins and minerals, especially chromium, needed for the glucose tolerance factor. The refining of sugar, flour or rice loses over 90 % of the chromium content.

Turning Glucose into Energy

Within each of our thirty trillion or so cells exist tiny energy factories called mitochondria. The mitochondria turn glucose into another chemical, pyruvic acid, in the process of which a small amount of energy is released, which can be used by the cell to carry out its work. If this step occurs without sufficient oxygen present, a by-product builds up called lactic acid. That's why the first time you do strenuous exercise using muscles you didn't even know you had, the next day your muscles ache. This is, in part, because you've made them work too hard without supplying enough oxygen, causing a build up of lactic acid crystals. The more you exercise, developing larger muscles, the less strain you put on the muscles and the more oxygen they can use. This is what aerobic exercise is all about - providing muscle cells with enough oxygen so they can work properly.

Pyruvic acid then gets turned into acetyl-coenzyme A, or AcoA for short. This substance is perhaps the most vital because if you're starved of glucose, for example when a marathon runner 'hits the wall', you can break down fat or protein to AcoA, and use this for energy. However it's rather inefficient so the body prefers to use carbohydrate for fuel.

From this point on oxygen is needed every step of the way. AcoA enters a series of chemical reactions known as the Krebs cycle, after its discoverer, Ernst Krebs, which separates off hydrogen molecules, which then meet oxygen and BANG! Energy is released. In fact over 90% of all our energy is derived in this final stage. The waste products are carbon dioxide, which we exhale, water, which goes to form urine,

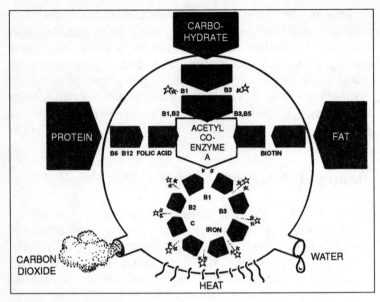

Figure 7 - Turning Food Into Energy

and heat. That's why we get hot when exercising, because muscle cells make lots of energy, so heat is created.

The Energy Nutrients

If you're thinking all you need to do is eat complex carbohydrates and keep breathing, that's only half the story. All these chemical reactions are carefully controlled by enzymes, themselves dependent on no less than eight vitamins and five minerals. Any shortage of these critical catalysts and your energy factories, the mitochondria, go out of tune. The result is inefficient energy production, a loss of stamina, highs and lows - or just lows.

The important vitamins are the B complex vitamins, every one essential for making energy. Glucose can't be turned into pyruvic acid without B1 and B3 (niacin). AcoA can't be formed without B1, B2, B3 and, most important of all, B5 (pantothenic acid). The Krebs cycle needs B1, B2 and B3 to do its job properly. Fats and proteins can't be used to make energy without B6, B12, folic acid or biotin.

Vitamins for Vitality

It used to be thought that as long as you ate a reasonable diet you'd get enough B vitamins. But studies have shown that long-term slight deficiencies gradually result in a depletion of these vitamins in cells, causing early warning signs of deficiency such as poor skin condition, anxiety, depression, mental confusion, irritability, but most of all, fatigue. Many people's diets fall short on these vital vitamins. The Booker Survey in 1985 showed that only one in ten people ate a diet that provided the Recommended Daily Allowance for B6 or folic acid. In one study at the Institute for Optimum Nutrition, a group of 82 volunteers, many of whom already had a 'well balanced diet' were assessed to calculate their optimal nutritional needs. All 82 were given extra B vitamins in supplement form, often in doses twenty times that of the RDA's. After six months 79% of participants reported a definite improvement in energy, 61% felt physically fitter and 60% had noticed an improvement in their mental alertness and memory.

Being water soluble, B vitamins are easily lost when foods are boiled in water, as well as being extremely sensitive to heat. The best natural sources are therefore fresh fruit, raw vegetables and wheatgerm. Seeds, nuts and wholegrains contain reasonable amounts, as do meat, fish, eggs and dairy produce. But these levels are reduced when the food is cooked or stored for a long time.

The minerals iron, calcium, magnesium, chromium and zinc are also vital for making energy. Calcium and magnesium are perhaps the most important because all muscle cells need an adequate supply of these to be able to contract and relax. A shortage of magnesium, so common in those who don't eat much fruit or vegetables, often results in muscle cramps, as the muscle is unable to relax.

But vitamins and minerals aren't all that's involved. The final stage before energy can be released is dependent on a special coenzyme, coenzyme Q (Co-Q). A vital link in the chain, Co-Q provides the spark together with oxygen, to keep our energy furnace burning.

The recent discovery that Co-Q is present in foods, that levels decline with age, and that cellular levels rise when supplements are taken, has led many nutritional scientists to suspect that Co-Q may be the missing link in the energy equation.

7

ARE YOU A STIMULANT ADDICT?

Sugar isn't the only chemical that alters blood sugar levels. So does caffeine, theobromine and theophylline, found in tea, coffee, chocolate, cola drinks and fizzy drinks with added caffeine.

Consumption of coffee, tea, sugar and chocolate are all associated with an increased risk of diabetes. In the short-term they may give a boost, but in the long-term high stimulant consumption can kill you prematurely. Try this simple experiment. Quit your intake of these stimulants for one month. Notice what happens on withdrawal. The more damage stimulants are doing to you the greater the withdrawal effect. (Fortunately, by eating slow-releasing carbohydrates and taking supplements withdrawal symptoms usually last no more than four days.) Then start again and notice what happens with your first tea, coffee, hit of sugar and chocolate. You'll experience what Hans Selye called the 'initial response' - in other words a true response to these powerful chemicals. A pounding head, hyperactive mind, fast heart beat, insomnia, followed by extreme drowsiness. Keep on the stimulants and you will adapt - that's phase 2. Keep doing this long enough and eventually you hit exhaustion - phase 3. This happens for everybody. The only variance is how long it will take you to get to the 'exhaustion' phase.

Recovery is not only possible, it's usually rapid. Most people feel substantially more energy and resistanceto stress within 30 days of quitting stimulants with nutritional support. Coffee, tea and chocolate are best to just quit. Decaffeinated coffee and tea still contains stimulants.

Allergy or Addiction?

Stimulants directly boost our energy and change our state of mind. They have their effect by putting the body into an 'emergency' state called the 'fight-flight' syndrome because the changes that occur seem to prepare us for action. The heart beat increases, breathing increases, muscles get less tired, and blood sugar levels rise, all helping get fuel to the cells to make more energy. This may sound great but in the long run it's not, because this extra energy comes at a price.

To begin with, after the burst of energy afforded by, say a cup of coffee, there is often a dip some hours later. With regular consumption more of the stimulant is required to produce the same 'up'. Meanwhile symptoms such as sleepiness, aggressiveness, depression, dizziness, excessive thirst, headaches and sweating may become more frequent. After a while the only noticeably good effect of the food or drink is that symptoms such as these temporarily go away. By now you're hooked.

Many people also become addicted to normal foods such as bread and dairy produce. This is often a sign of food allergy. This means that, when a particular food is eaten, the immune system reacts, affecting both the body and the brain. Food allergies can trigger a whole host of symptoms from hyperactivity to depression, facial puffiness, bloating, blocked nose, headaches, sleepiness, skin problems and so on. The most common foods to cause allergic reactions are wheat and milk.

One of the strange signs of a food allergy is a craving for the food itself. For some people, provided they eat enough of their allergy frequently enough, symptoms can be 'masked' or suppressed. These people often feel worse in the morning, when they haven't eaten for a number of hours, or after a couple of days without their allergic food. But most people feel worse after consuming the substance to which they're allergic. Yet this doesn't stop them craving it.

Whether a stimulant or a food allergy, it isn't so difficult to become hooked on substances that alter how we feel. On top of that we develop psychological habits. Giving yourself chocolate, for example, when you're down; or bingeing on biscuits when you're burnt out. Even if you know these things are bad for you, how do you break the habit?

Kicking the Habit

Top of the list of food addiction is tea and coffee. Coffee contains three stimulants - caffeine, theobromine and theophylline. Although caffeine is the strongest, theophylline is known to disturb normal sleep patterns and theobromine has a similar effect to caffeine, although it is present in much smaller amounts in coffee. So decaffeinated coffee isn't exactly stimulant free.

A lot of coffee is definitely bad for you. High coffee consumers have a greater risk of cancer of the pancreas and, if pregnant, a higher risk of birth defects [1,2]. Coffee also stops minerals being absorbed. The amount of iron absorbed reduces to one third if coffee is drunk with a meal [3]. Coffee, taken during exams, has a negative effect on performance.

More controversial are the effects of small amounts of coffee. As a nutritionist I have seen many people cleared of minor health problems such as tiredness and headaches just from stopping drinking two or three coffees a day. The best way to find out what effect it has on you is to quit for a trial period of two weeks. You may get withdrawal symptoms for up to three days. These reflect how addicted you've become. After that, if you begin to feel perky and your health improves that is a good indication that you're better off without coffee. The most popular alternatives are Caro Extra, made with roasted barley, chicory and rye, dandelion coffee (Symingtons or Lanes) or herb teas.

Tea is the great British addiction. A strong cup of tea contains as much caffeine as a weak cup of coffee and is certainly addictive. Tea also contains tannin which interferes with the absorption of vital minerals such as iron and zinc. Like coffee, drinking too much tea is also associated with a number of health problems including an increased risk of stomach ulcers. Particularly addictive is Earl Grey tea containing bergamot, itself a stimulant. If you're addicted to tea and can't get going without a cuppa it may be time to stop for two weeks and see how you feel. The best tasting alternatives are Rooibosch tea (red bush tea) with milk, herb and fruit teas. Drinking very weak tea irregularly is unlikely to be a problem.

Chocoholism

Chocolate is full of sugar. It also contains cocoa as its major active ingredient. Cocoa provides significant quantities of the stimulant theobromine, whose action is similar although not as strong as caffeine. Theobromine is also obtained in cocoa drinks like hot chocolate. Being high in sugar and stimulants, plus its delicious taste, it's easy to become a chocoholic. The best way to quit the habit is to have one month with NO chocolate. Instead you can eat healthy 'sweets' from health food shops. My favourites are Sunflower bars and Karriba bars. After a month you will have lost the craving for chocolate.

Coke Abuse

Certain cola and other fizzy drinks contain between 5 and 7mg of caffeine which is a quarter of that found in a weak cup of coffee. In addition, these drinks are often high in sugar and colourings and their net stimulant effect can be considerable. Check the ingredients and stay away from drinks containing caffeine, chemicals or colourings.

Habit Breakers

Changing any food habit causes stress so it is best not to quit everything in one go. So a good strategy is to avoid something for a month and then see how you feel. One way to greatly reduce the cravings for foods you've got hooked on is by having an excellent diet. Since all stimulants affect blood sugar levels you can keep yours even by always having something substantial for breakfast such as an oat based breakfast or unsweetened live yoghurt with banana, ground sesame seeds and wheatgerm, or an egg, and frequent snacks of fresh fruit. The worst thing you can do is go for hours without eating. Research from Columbia University in New York suggests that eating a highly alkaline-forming diet can reduce craving for cigarettes and alcohol [4]. This means eating lots of fresh vegetables and fruit. These high fibre foods also help to keep your blood sugar level even.

Vitamins and minerals are important too because they help to regulate your blood sugar level, and hence your appetite. They also minimise the withdrawal effects of stimulants and the symptoms of food allergy. The key nutrients are vitamin C, the B complex vitamins, especially vitamin B6, and the minerals calcium and magnesium. Fresh fruit and vegetables provide significant amounts of vitamin C and B vitamins, while vegetables and seeds, such as sunflower and sesame, are good sources of calcium and magnesium. For maximum effect, however, it is best to supplement these nutrients as well as eating foods rich in them. I recommend a high strength multivitamin containing at least 100mg of vitamin B6, plus 2,000mg per day of vitamin C and some calcium and magnesium (see Chapter 21).

8

SOLVING THE STRESS SYNDROME

But if sugar, sweet foods and stimulants are so bad for us, why do we like them so much? The answer to this simple question provides the answer to probably a third of all western diseases. The answer lies deeply rooted in our biological ancestry. Whether you like the idea or not, we human beings belong to the family 'primates'. Like our ancestors we are equipped with certain instincts, inborn programming for survival. One of these, the enjoyment of sweetness, is probably there to protect us from nature's more poisonous food. Almost anything sweet is safe. Fruits are safe, berries are safe. It's a good rule. For the plant kingdom it also makes sense, because when animals eat plants the seeds are deposited with a pile of manure - a good start in life!

But mankind, being smarter than its ancestors, learnt to extract and concentrate the source of sweetness until, in the 20th century, we are left with pure, white and deadly sucrose - sugar.

That's half the story. The other half is all about stress. All primates also have a powerful system for coping with stress. It's called the fight-flight syndrome, because it is designed to help you get up a tree if you're hunted, run faster if you're hunting and heal wounds rapidly if you're fighting. Even though today's stresses are more likely to be mortgages or demands at work, the same system operates. For example, if you're frustrated because you're stuck in a traffic jam your blood still coagulates faster, just in case you're wounded! Digestion also slows down to channel biological activity to increasing the supply of glucose to muscle cells for extra energy. We can't stop it happening - and the evidence suggests we don't want to stop stress even if we could.

Although we all complain about stress, could it be that there is a part of us that actually craves it? After all, given spare time, how many of us avoid stress? Instead we take part in or watch violent contact sports, drive around in fast cars, go skiing or do other such dangerous activities, and even if we do put our feet up, it's usually to watch the news, or the 2.5 murders that happen every night on our TV sets. Meanwhile the children are playing space invaders or watching horror videos! Have you heard about Peter's Principle? It identifies that people like to get promoted in work to their level of incompetence! We strive for more pressure, more challenge. If we can't get it we turn to nutritional stressors like coffee, tea, chocolate, cigarettes or drugs. Consider the case of a rich housewife who repeatedly shoplifts. Such cases appear in the courts every year. Money isn't the motive. It's the thrill - the effects of the stress hormone, adrenalin.

We, like our ancestors, are addicted to adrenalin. But unlike our ancestors we don't fight, we don't hunt and we don't run. Our stresses no longer require a physical response. Yet for our ancestors and other primates it is the physical response that uses up the extra sugar that pours into our bloodstream. For us, we have to restore balance by producing more insulin, which lowers blood sugar levels by transporting the glucose into the cells, where it is converted to glycogen or fat. In fact, modern man produces gallons more insulin than his ancestors. With this context it is hardly surprising that diabetes, a disease in which the pancreas effectively stops producing insulin, is on the increase and accounts for 17% of all deaths.

Ultimately there is only one way out of the vicious circle of using adrenal stimulants to give you short bursts of energy. That is stop, or at least reduce, nutritional stressors. If, at the same time, you replace those nutrients that are used up by continual stress any 'withdrawal' effects are minimal and recovery to full vitality is fastest.

The Chemistry of Stress

Whatever thoughts you have about stress the reality is that body chemistry fundamentally changes every time a person reacts stressfully. Stress starts in the mind. We perceive a situation as requiring our immediate attention - a young child getting too close to the road, a car getting too close to us, a hostile reaction from another, a financial crisis, an impossible deadline. Rapid signals stimulate the adrenal glands on top of the kidneys in the small of the back, to produce adrenalin. Within seconds your heart is pounding, your breathing changes, stores of glucose are released into the blood, the muscles tense, the eyes dilate, even the blood thickens.

What, you might ask, has all this got to do with calling the bank manager? The answer is very little, however before the days of overdraft facilities most stresses required a physical response. That's what adrenalin does. It gets you ready to fight or take flight. The average adrenalin rush of a commuter stuck in a traffic jam is enough to keep them running for a mile. That's how much glucose is released, mainly by breaking down glycogen held in muscles and the liver. The hormones insulin, glucagon and GTF all swing into action to balance blood sugar. All this is happening as a result of a stressful thought.

Where, you might wonder, does all this extra energy and increased alertness come from? The answer is by diverting energy from the body's normal repair and maintenance jobs such as digesting, cleansing, and rejuvenating. So, every moment you spend in stress the ageing process of your body speeds up. It's stressful even thinking about it. But the effects of prolonged stress are even more insidious than that. Imagine your pituitary, adrenals, pancreas and liver perpetually pumping out hormones to control blood sugar that you don't even need day in, day out. Like a car driven too fast the body goes out of balance and parts start to wear out.

DHEA - The Anti-Ageing Adrenal Hormone

One of the more reliable indicators of adrenal exhaustion is the level of an adrenal hormone called DHEA, an abbreviation for 'dehydroepiandrosterone'. DHEA not only helps control stress, it also maintains proper mineral balance, helps control the production of sex hormones and build lean body mass while reducing fat tissue. Increased levels of DHEA, nick-named the anti-ageing hormone, have many benefits associated with youth. Levels start to decline after the age of twenty, especially in who live in a state of prolonged stress. DHEA levels can be measured in blood and in saliva and low levels can be boosted by DHEA supplementation, together with stress management through diet, exercise and lifestyle changes.

Addicted to stress

As a consequence of prolonged stress your energy level drops, you lose concentration, get confused, suffer from bouts of 'brain fag', fall asleep after meals, get irritable, freak out, can't sleep, can't wake up, sweat too much, get headaches... sounds familiar? In an attempt to regain control most people turn to stimulants to keep them going.

Of course, you can't live like this forever, so most people burn out and have to head for the beach to recover. Yet as they wait in the airport what could be a better way to relax than read a fiction novel? The back page says 'murder, mystery, greed, lust, gripping suspense'. Sounds good. Then, after two blissful hours of engrossment in murder, mystery and intrigue on the beach it's time for some excitement - windsurfing, waterskiing, something exciting. What is it we're looking for? In an interview with Evel Knievel in the cockpit of his rocket 'bike' an interviewer asked "Why do you do it?" Evil replied to the effect that "there is a moment when I'm flying through the air of absolute peace." He closed the hatch, pressed the button and seconds later the rocket slammed into the side of the Grand Canyon. I first heard this story in the introduction to a meditation course. The speaker concluded by saying "There must be an easier way than this." The point is that most people become addicted to stress, and to the highly physiologically addictive cocktail of chemical 'uppers' and 'downers'. The deluded mind convinces them that this level of excitement is the best that life has to offer.

Energy Consumers

Yet, in a very real sense all stressors and stimulants consume our energy. The 'high' is literally energy leaving the system, like the wave that breaks and seems, for a few seconds, to be full of energy. A few seconds later there is no wave at all, the energy is gone. Oscar Ichazo, in an article on drug abuse, says "Drugs (all of them) can be characterised as 'energy consumers', consuming energy at a rate much greater than our natural ability to replace it [1]. As drugs burn all our accumulated vitality in short periods of time, the brief exaltation is inevitably followed by depletion of vital energy, felt as the 'down', the depressant effect of drugs. Nothing can replace a natural, clean body capable of producing natural and clean vital energy." He rates the drugs most damaging to our vital energy in this order: First alcohol, then heroine and opiates, tobacco, cocaine, barbiturates, anti-depressants, amphetamines, marijuana and caffeine sources.

But what does it mean to 'consume energy'? Well, it literally means that body cells are starved of fuel nutrients, like glucose, and catalyst nutrients, like B vitamins which drive the enzyme systems necessary to release energy from fuel nutrients. The nutrients necessary to make messenger molecules like neurotransmitters, or carrier molecules like insulin, are also depleted. The list is long - eight B vitamins, vitamin C, co-enzyme Q, chromium, zinc, magnesium, calcium, manganese, choline, and the amino acids glutamine, tyrosine, tryptophan, phenylalanine and others. What this means is that every moment you spend in a stressful state you are using up nutrients. Consider this. Have you ever had a massage, after which you felt like a whole load of muscular tension had gone? Every single muscle cell that you hold in tension, often for decades even when you are asleep, is consuming energy, B vitamins, vitamin C, calcium and magnesium to name a few just to stay in a state of tension. If you could relax all the muscles in your body think how much you'd save in nutritional supplements! Conservative estimates suggest that you double your need for vitamins in a 'stress' state.

The Energy Equation

If you want to maximise your available mental and physical energy, rather than burning out, from a nutritional point of view the message is simple:

1   Eat foods that release their 'fuel' slowly.
2   Ensure optimal intakes of all essential nutrients.
3   Avoid stimulants and depressants.
4   Avoid unnecessary stress.

The result of doing this is a guaranteed increase in available energy that helps us to cope with the stresses and strains of life. The optimum nutrition approach is both a way of breaking energy consuming patterns that keep depleting us, and regenerating energy for breaking the mental habits that initiate a stress response in the first place.

9

BRAIN ALLERGIES

Lucretius said, around 50 BC "One man's meat is another man's poison." Of course, this is many people's experience. Some foods suit and some don't. Some days you feel good and some days you don't. Often, there is the awareness that it may be connected to what you eat, but the riddle isn't easy to decipher.

Based on fifteen years clinical experience I believe the majority of people have food allergies or intolerances. For most the symptoms are minor. For a minority they conform to the classic 'IgE allergy' where there is an instant reaction to, for example, shell fish. The majority, however, seem to suffer from delayed food sensitivity, in which the reaction occurs anywhere from 2 to 48 hours later. This kind of reaction is now thought to involve a different kind of immune antibody which reacts to an accumulation of allergy-provoking food molecules.

So what's all this got to do with mental health? Most food allergies provoke mental and emotional changes. This is an idea which has been resisted by conventional allergists, but has been borne out both by clinical tests and by scientific analysis.

Brain cells 'communicate' through the action of neurotransmitters. This is the whole foundation of a chemical model of mental health. Yet brain cells are not unique in being able to communicate in this way. The body's immune cells in the digestive tract, blood and body tissue also have receptors to many neurotransmitters. Scientists are beginning to discover there's a lot of conversations going on between the brain and nervous system, the immune system and endocrine system. You could call the study of these interactions 'psycho-neuro-immuno-endocrinology'! In truth, this is a highly fertile ground in medical science today as we gradually learn that the boundaries between mind and body are extremely fuzzy. Simultaneously, we are discovering a much closer connection between allergies and mental health (discussed in depth in Chapter 19). To understand this connection it's necessary to understand what an allergy is in the first place.

Mental Symptoms related to Food Allergy

Anxiety	Attention Deficit
Depression	Headaches
Hyperactivity	Insomnia
Learning Disorders	Tension-Fatigue Syndrome
Delusions	Dyslexia
Epilepsy	Hallucinations
Memory Loss	Premenstrual Syndrome

What is Allergy?

The classic definition of an allergy is 'any idiosyncratic reaction where the immune system is clearly involved'. The immune system, which is the body's defence system, has the ability to produce 'markers' for substances it doesn't like. The classic marker is an antibody called IgE (immunoglobulin type E). These attach themselves to 'mast cells' in the body. When the offending food, called an allergen, complexes with its specific IgE antibody, the IgE molecule triggers the mast cell to release granules containing histamine and other chemicals that cause the symptoms of classic allergy - skin rashes, hayfever, rhinitis, sinusitis, asthma, eczema and severe food allergies to, for example, shellfish or peanuts, causing immediate gastrointestinal upsets or swelling in the face or throat. All these reactions are immediate, severe inflammatory reactions and are known as Type 1 allergic reactions.

The emerging view now is that most allergies and intolerances, diplomatically called by some 'idiosyncratic' reactions, are not IgE based. There is a new school of thought and a new generation of allergy tests, designed to detect intolerances not based on IgE antibody reactions, but probably involving another marker, known as IgG. According to Dr James Braly, director of Immuno Laboratories, which developed the IgG ELISA test, "Food allergy is not rare, nor are the effects limited to the air passages, the skin and digestive tract. Most food allergies are delayed reactions, taking anywhere from an hour to three days to show themselves, and are therefore much harder to detect. Delayed food allergy appears to be simply the inability of your digestive tract to prevent large quantities of partially digested and undigested food from entering the bloodstream."

This is not a new idea. Since the 1950's pioneering allergists such as Dr Theron Randolph, Herbert Rinkel, Dr Arthur Coca, and, more recently, Dr William Philpott and Dr Marshall Mandel, have written about delayed sensitivities causing far-reaching effects on all systems of the body, including the mind. These were the 'heretics' of classic allergy theory, however their ideas are now being proven right with advances in scientific methods for determining other types of immune reactions.

IgG antibodies were first discovered in the 1960's and are still considered reasonably irrelevant by some conventional allergists The problem, say the critics, is that most people have many IgG based reactions to foods without apparently suffering from allergies. The IgG antibodies may serve as 'tags' but don't initiate a reaction. However, say the advocates, a large build-up of IgG antibodies to a particular food indicates a chronic long-term sensitivity, or food intolerance. It is now well established that many, if not the majority of food intolerances, do not produce immediate symptoms, but have a delayed, accumulative effect. This, of course, makes them hard to detect by

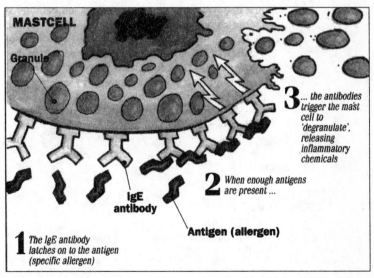

Figure 9 - IgE, meeting allergen, and triggering mast cell to degranulate, causing reaction.

observation. Dr Hill, researching in Australia, found that the majority of food sensitive children reacted after 2 or more hours to foods. In contrast IgE reactions are immediate, suggesting that a build up of IgG antibodies may be a primary factor in food sensitivity.

According to Dr Jonathan Brostoff, consultant in medical immunology at the Middlesex Hospital Medical School, certain ingested substances can cause the release of histamine, now known to have profound effects on mental health, and invoke classical allergic symptoms without involving IgE. These include lectins (in peanuts), shellfish, tomatoes, pork, alcohol, chocolate, pineapple, papaya, buckwheat, sunflower, mango and mustard. He also thinks it is possible that undigested proteins could directly affect mast cells in the gut, which contain histamine, causing the classic symptoms of allergy.

One common reaction, known as Type 3 allergy, is said to occur when there is a substantial production of antibodies (mainly IgG) in response to an allergen in the blood. This results in immune complexes. "It is the sheer weight of numbers that causes a problem," says Brostoff. "These immune complexes are like litter going round in the bloodstream." The litter is cleaned up by cells, principally neutrophils, that act like vacuum cleaners. Cytotoxic allergy tests are designed to measure changes in number, size and activity of neutrophils when exposed to certain foods, to determine possible food allergies.

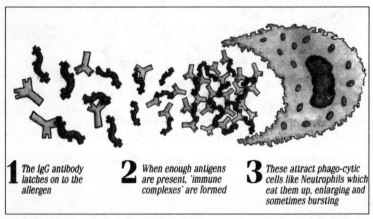

1 The IgG antibody latches on to the allergen

2 When enough antigens are present, 'immune complexes' are formed

3 These attract phago-cytic cells like Neutrophils which eat them up, enlarging and sometimes bursting

Figure 10 - IgG complexes attracting neutrophil degranulation

How IgG and IgE antibodies relate is another area of debate. Allergy specialist Dr Braly has seen a number of patients who have both an immediate and delayed reaction to a food, suggesting a link between the immediate short-term IgE type reaction and the delayed IgG reaction. Dr Anders Hoy from Denmark suspects that long-term build up of IgG to a particular food might switch to an IgE type sensitivity, causing immediate allergic response.

IgG Allergy Testing - The New Generation?

The first type of tests to move away from measuring immediate IgE reactions were the 'cytotoxic' tests, which means 'toxic to cells'. These tests observe changes to immune cells called neutrophils which come along and clean up 'immune complexes' caused by antibody-antigen reactions. Cytotoxic tests are thought to reflect IgG sensitivity.

The state-of-the-art for measuring IgG sensitivity is a relatively new technique, developed over the last eight years, involving a method known as ELISA. ELISA testing for IgG sensitivity claims more reproducible and reliable results than cytotoxic testing, and indeed samples tested by both methods are not often consistent in results. One possibility is that these tests measure different types of reactions. Another is that one or more of the tests is unreliable.

Allergy or Indigestion?

Dr Hoy, who is a convert to the new ELISA IgG testing, believes that 'healthy' foods cause allergic reaction because they are not properly digested. "If food is not broken down into small molecules you start producing IgG antibodies. The immune cells have to work hard to produce masses of IgGs, reducing the immune system's capacity for fighting infection." says Hoy, who has observed that people with pronounced IgG reactions produce little stomach acid, which would lead to poor indigestion and a greater chance of allergy. Whether this is a cause or effect of allergy isn't clear, however, for many allergy sufferers low hydrochloric acid production is part of the picture.

Both Dr Hoy and Dr Braly prescribe the same remedy - avoid foods that provoke an IgG reaction to lessen the load on the immune system, and then focus on improving digestion. Dr Braly has found zinc deficiency to be extremely common among allergy sufferers. Zinc is not only needed to digest all protein, it's also essential for the production of hydrochloric acid in the stomach. Certain foods, he says, are inherently difficult to digest, the worst being gluten in wheat. Wheat and dairy are Britain's top two allergy provoking foods.

He also suspects that many allergy sufferers may have excessively 'leaky' gut walls, allowing undigested proteins to enter the food and cause reactions. Consumption of alcohol, frequent use of aspirin, deficiency in essential fatty acids or a gastrointestinal infection or infestation, such as candidiasis, are all possible contributors to leaky gut syndrome that need to be corrected to reduce a person's sensitivity to foods.

Cross-Reactions

Another contributor to food sensitivity is exposure to inhalants that provoke a reaction. For example, it is well known that, when the pollen count is high more people suffer from hayfever in polluted areas that rural areas despite lower pollen counts in cities. It is thought that exposure to exhaust fumes makes a pollen-allergic more sensitive. Whether this is simply because their immune system is weakened from dealing with the pollution and therefore less able to cope with the additional pollen insult, or due to some kind of 'cross-reaction' is not known. In the US, where ragweed sensitivity is common, a cross-reaction with bananas has been reported. In other words, one sensitivity sensitises you to another. A similar cross-reaction may occur with pollen, wheat and milk for hayfever sufferers.

The emerging view, shared by an increasing number of allergy specialists is that food sensitivity is a multi-factorial phenomenon possibly involving poor nutrition, pollution, digestive problems and over-exposure to certain foods. Removing the foods may help the sufferer recover, but other factors need to be dealt with in order to have a major impact on long-term food intolerance.

How Long to Avoid?

Just how long allergens have to be avoided is another open-ended question. Foods that invoke an IgE type, immediate and pronounced reaction may need to be avoided for life. The 'memory' of IgE antibodies is long-term. In contrast, B-cells that produce IgG antibodies have a half-life of six weeks. That means that there are half as many six weeks later. The 'memory' of these antibodies is short-term and, within six months, there is unlikely to be any residual 'memory' of reaction to a food that's been avoided. While a six month avoidance may be ideal, Hoy and Braly report good results after as little as a month. Another option, after a strict one month avoidance, is to 'rotate' foods so that an IgG sensitive food is only eaten every 4 days. This reduces the build up of allergen-antibody complexes and reduces the chances of an intolerance. Foods such as wheat and milk are probably best eaten infrequently.

The Top Ten Allergies

The protein molecules in food cause the majority of allergic reactions particularly those foods we eat most frequently. Top of the list is wheat, probably because it contains a substance called gliadin which is irritable to the gut wall. Gliadin is contained in gluten, a sticky protein that allows pockets to form when reacted with yeast, which is how bread is made. Eating a lot of wheat products isn't good for anyone, especially if you've developed an allergy. The connection between wheat allergy and mental health is well established (see Chapter 19).

Dairy produce produces allergic reactions in many people. This includes cheese and yoghurt. Some people can tolerate goat's or sheep's milk but not cow's milk. The symptoms are very varied but often include blocked nose, frequent 'colds', bloating and indigestion, 'thick' head, fatigue and headaches. Other foods that can cause allergic reactions include oranges, eggs, other grains yeast containing foods, shellfish, nuts, beef, pork and onions. Some people also develop allergies to tea and coffee, while alcohol, which irritates the gut wall and makes it more leaky, often increases allergic sensitivity.

If you have a history of infantile colic, eczema, asthma, ear infections or hayfever, have seasonal allergies, frequent rapid colds, have daily mood swings or function better off certain foods you may have a food intolerance. Often it's best to see a nutrition consultant who can decipher the likely culprits from your symptoms and eating patterns, advise you on tests, should they prove necessary, and help you correct digestive problems that increase your allergic potential. Also read Chapter 19, which explores the link between mental illness and allergy.

10

SMART NUTRIENTS

Most people believe that intelligence is something you're born with and nothing you do can change it. Despite the fact that numerous studies have shown increases in IQ scores, mental performance, memory, concentration and problem solving through changes in nutrition, the idea that what you eat affects the brain is still vigorously resisted. The brain and nervous system, our mental 'hardware', is made out of nutrients. The chemical messengers in the brain, neurotransmitters, are also derived from nutrients. Can we improve our mental performance or is intelligence something your born with, never to change?

There are clearly limits imposed to the hardware by genetic inheritance and the available nutrients during critical periods of brain development, which may define the limits to one's ability to develop intelligence. But changes in the nutritional status of an individual have been clearly demonstrated to improve mental performance, as have strategies for facilitating learning and memory. So, if you want to be smarter what should you eat?

Smart Food

The brain and nervous system uses up more than half of available nutrients supplied during foetal development. Once born the brain continues to need an abundant supply of nutrients. Particularly important are the essential fatty acids and phospholipids which form part of the structure of brain cell membranes. Low levels of essential fatty acids equate with lower levels of intelligence. This is thought to be the reason why breast-fed babies, by the age of seven, have higher IQ scores. Breast milk contains DHA, an essential fatty acid essential for brain development. The richest dietary source of DHA is fish. Phospholipids are also found in abundant supply in fish.

Probably the most important phospholipid is phosphatidyl choline

68

How to BOOST Your Brain Power

1   Reduce your intake of stimulants - coffee, tea, chocolate, cola, sugar and refined foods.
2   Ensure optimum nutrition through diet and taking a high dose multivitamin and mineral supplement.
3   Supplement smart nutrients: pantothenic acid 100-500mg per day; choline 500-1,000mg; DMAE 100-500mg per day; pyroglutamate 250-750mg per day.
4   Minimise your exposure to pollution - and cigarettes.

which also supplies the brain nutrient choline, needed to make acetylcholine, a vital neurotransmitter for memory, control of sensory input signals, and muscular control. Deficiency in acetylcholine results in poor memory, lethargy, decreased dreaming and a dry mouth. This is thought to be one of the major causes of dementia, which affects one in every five people over the age of 80. In animal studies, giving phosphatidyl choline increases brain levels of acetylcholine and improves memory [1]. Some researchers believe that an inability to make use of phospholipids such as choline may underlie diseases such as Alzheimers [2].

Acetylcholine - The Memory Molecule

Acetylcholine is made by the action of an enzyme, dependent on vitamin B5, acting on choline. The combination of vitamin B5 and choline has proven effective in enhancing memory and mental performance. Choline, although not classified as such, may be an essential nutrient. Recent studies have shown that it is essential to have some in your diet for the liver to function normally. [3] The best supplemental source of choline is lecithin which also supply phospholipids. Lecithin is an emulsifier that is even used in some foods. All health food stores stock it, either as capsules or granules. The granules are best and can be sprinkled on food. However, not all lecithin is the same. Look at the label before you buy, and make sure the product contains more than 30% phosphatidyl choline.

However, one problem with supplementing any form of choline is

BRAIN CELL COMMUNICATION

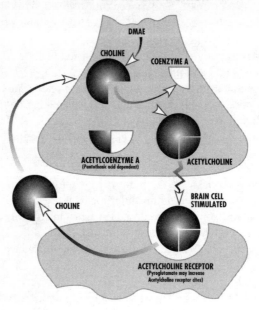

Figure 11- Acetylcholine

that it doesn't readily cross the blood brain barrier into brain cells, which is why large quantities, around a tablespoon a day of lecithin granules, are needed to have an effect. Another nutrient found in fish, and particularly rich in anchovies and sardines, is DMAE (dimethylaminoethanol) which passes easily into the brain, and can be converted into choline to make acetylcholine. DMAE has been shown to elevate mood, improve memory, increase intelligence, increase physical energy and extend the life of laboratory animals. One of the pioneers of DMAE therapy, Dr Carl Pfeiffer, found it to be an excellent slow acting stimulant - an alternative to anti-depressants. It is now prescribed, often under the name Deaner or Deanol, for learning problems, hyperactivity, reading and speech difficulties and behavioural problems in children and is currently being researched for its effects on extending lifespan. As one person on DMAE said "I am more awake when I'm awake, and more sound asleep when I'm asleep.

Not only does my memory improve, but I have an easier time day dreaming when I want to , and concentrating on real world tasks when I want to."

Nootropics

The buzz word in brain enhancement is 'nootropics'. These are substances derived from an amino acid called pyroglutamate which is found in fruit and vegetables. The discovery that the brain and cerebrospinal fluid contains large amounts of pyroglutamate led to its investigation as an essential brain nutrient. Doctors prescribe nootropics to millions of people every year for memory deficit problems. Their basic effect is to improve learning, memory consolidation and memory retrieval with no toxicity or side-effects. One extraordinary finding was that nootropics promote the flow of information between the right and left hemispheres of the brain. This is thought to be a possible reason why nootropics have proven helpful in the treatment of dyslexia. A study, published in 1988 by Dr Pilch and colleagues, suggests that nootropics may increase the number of acetylcholine receptors in the brain. Older mice were given piracetam, a pyroglutamate derivative, for two weeks. The researchers found that these older mice had 30-40% higher density of receptors than before. This suggests that pyroglutamate-like molecules do not only maximise mental performance but may also have a regenerative effect on the nervous system.

Synergy - Why 1+1=4

The effects of enhancing mental performance through supplementation of 'smart nutrients' such as phosphatidyl choline, pantothenic acid, DMAE and pyroglutamate are likely to be far greater when taken in combination than individually. In one study in 1981, a team of researchers led by Raymond Bartus gave choline and piracetam, a pyroglutamate derivative, to aged lab rats noted for age-related memory decline. They found that "rats given the piracetam/choline combination exhibited (memory) retention scores several times better than those with piracetam alone." They found that half the dose was needed when piracetam and choline were combined.

The combined use of vitamins and minerals has also proven

beneficial for schoolchildren in improving mental performance. Four studies have shown significant increases in IQ scores as a result of supplementing 'optimal' doses of vitamins and minerals.The first study to test the overall effects of vitamins and minerals on mental performance was carried out by Gwillym Roberts, a schoolteacher and nutritionist from ION, and David Benton, a psychologist from Swansea University College, who put 60 schoolchildren onto a special multivitamin and mineral supplement designed to ensure an optimal intake of key nutrients.[4] Without their knowledge half these children were placed on a placebo. On analysing the diets of these schoolchildren a significant minority were getting less than the RDA level of at least one nutrient. After eight months on the supplements the non-verbal IQ's in those taking the supplements had risen by over 10 points! No changes were seen in those on the placebos, or a control group of students who had not taken any supplements or placebos.

Clearly, supplements had an effect but the questions raised were: who benefits and why, which nutrients are important at which levels and how long does it take to get an effect? To answer some of these questions 615 schoolchildren in California were assigned to either a placebo group or one of three 'supplement' groups given approximately 50%, 100% and 200% of the US RDAs for vitamins and minerals. After one month only the 200% RDA group had significantly higher IQ scores than the placebo group. After three months, all supplement groups had higher IQ scores than the placebo group, with the 100% RDA having the highest, and statistically significant, increase. Of this group 45% had an increase in IQ of 15 or more points, compared to the average increase of 4.4 points.

Other studies of children with learning difficulties, discussed fully in Chapter 20, have had promising results. In one study by Dr Michael Colgan compared the results achieved by children with learning difficulties attending a remedial learning course with or without multinutrients. Those given multinutrients had an increase in IQ of 17.9 points and an increase in reading age equivalent to 1.8 years, compared to those not on supplements of 1.1 years and an 8.4 point shift in IQ. Similar controlled studies have yet to be carried out on adults. However, it is likely that daily supplementation with multinutrients may increase the effects of taking in specific nutrients for enhancing brain function.

Brain Circulation

Ginko Biloba is one of the oldest species of trees, dating back some 300 million years. Extracts have been used by the Chinese for thousands of years to improve mental performance. To date some 40 studies have been published, showing that gingko does improve blood flow throughout the body and in the brain. It is a powerful antioxidant and improves the brain's ability to use glucose and hence derive energy. Some consider it to be a nootropic and certainly there's enough evidence to back its authenticity as a smart nutrient.

Other powerful antioxidants, such as vitamins A, beta-carotene, C, E, proanthocyanidins, lipoic acid, melatonin and others, may also contribute to maximum mental performance.

The Brain Drain

While 'good' chemicals, nutrients, can improve mental function, 'bad' chemicals can and do reduce your intelligence. Alcohol is a prime example. Coffee, while commonly thought to improve concentration, actually diminishes it. A number of studies have shown that the ability to remember lists of words is made worse by caffeine. According to one researcher "Caffeine may have a deleterious effect on the rapid processing of ambiguous or confusing stimuli", which sounds like a description of modern living! The combination of caffeine and alcohol slows reaction time and, in one study, made subjects more drunk than alcohol alone. Caffeine is present in coffee, tea, chocolate, Lucozade, cola drinks and guarana. A diet high in sugar and refined carbohydrates is another factor that reduces intelligence ratings. Research at the Massachusetts Institute of Technology found 26% difference in IQ between children with very high or very low refined sugar intakes.

Heavy metals such as lead, cadmium and aluminium accumulate in the brain and have been clearly demonstrated to worsen intelligence, concentration, memory and impulse control. Therefore, keeping pollution to a minimum, which includes not smoking, is also a prerequisite to boosting your brain power.

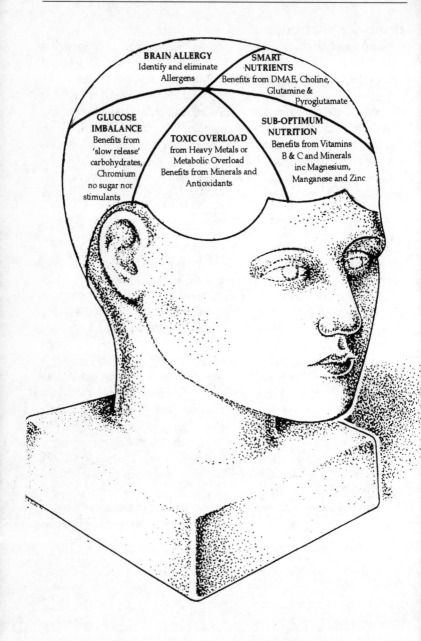

BRAIN ALLERGY
Identify and eliminate
Allergens

SMART NUTRIENTS
Benefits from DMAE, Choline,
Glutamine &
Pyroglutamate

GLUCOSE IMBALANCE
Benefits from
'slow release'
carbohydrates,
Chromium
no sugar nor
stimulants

TOXIC OVERLOAD
from Heavy Metals or
Metabolic Overload
Benefits from Minerals and
Antioxidants

SUB-OPTIMUM NUTRITION
Benefits from Vitamins
B & C and Minerals
inc Magnesium,
Manganese and Zinc

About the Author

Dr Carl Pfeiffer dedicated his life to establishing the link between nutrition and mental health. Having researched biochemical causes of mental illness since the 1930's he turned his attention exclusively to nutrition in the 50's after having a massive heart attack from which he was expected to live no more than ten years. During the following years he discovered the importance of vitamin B6 and zinc in the treatment of schizophrenia and pioneered research into zinc and

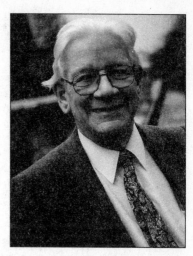

1909 - 1989

other micro-nutrients. He also identified two causes of mental illness: the genetic overproduction of histamine; and heavy metal toxicity; devising effective nutritional strategies to correct them.

In 1971 he founded the Princeton Bio Center in New Jersey, which continues to provide effective nutritional treatments to thousands of people suffering from mental illness and other conditions. His classic book, *Mental and Elemental Nutrients*, continues to inspire people to move towards optimum nutrition.

Rightly considered to have been the world's foremost authority on nutrition and mental illness, the significance of much of his work is yet to be fully realised.

This book is one of the last contributions of this great scientist. In the spirit of his pioneering work I (Patrick Holford) have revised, updated and expanded the original text to incorporate the new research that strengthens Dr Pfeiffer's conviction that mental illness can, in many cases, be successfully treated using nutritional therapy. Chapters 11, 12, 16, and 21 to 27 represent new material not present in the original manuscript he left for publication.

Contents

Foreword by Gwynneth Hemmings   80

Part 3 - Mental Illness - Not all in the mind

11 Understanding Mental Illness   82
    What is Mental Illness?   82
    Who Suffers?   83

12 Mental Illness - The Nutrition Connection   91
    Four Pillars of Mental Health   92
    Psychoanalysis or Neuroanalysis?   94

Part 4 - Mental Illness - The Modern Approach

13 The Modern Classification of Mental Illness   100

14 Overcoming Depression   102

15 Conquering Fears, Phobias & Hallucinations   108

16 Niacin Therapy - a Cure for Schizophrenia?   113

17 Pyroluria - the Zinc Link   118

18 Hypoglycemia - Over Stressed or   129
    Under Nourished

19 The Allergy Connection   135

20 Autism, Learning Difficulties & Dyslexia   145

21 Attention Deficit Disaster   149

22 Crime - Nourishment or Punishment?   156

23 Beating Addictions   162

24 Eating Disorders and Anorexia   168

25 Preventing Premature Senility   175

26 Solving Sleeping Problems   179

27 Fits, Convulsions, Epilepsy   182

28 Mood Swings & Manic Depression   184

29 Getting off Drugs   190

Part 5 - Action Plan For Mental Health

30 Finding Help & Staying out of Hospital   194

31 Diet & Supplements for Mental Health   196

32 Mental Health & Illness - The Nutrition Connection   208

Directory of Supplement Companies   199

Useful Addresses and Recommended Reading   200

Index   202

See reverse front for Contents of Chapters 1 to 10 on Mental Health - The Nutrition Connection

Foreword

The Chinese have a saying 'Disease enters through the mouth.' Yet it appears that many doctors do not like this concept. To consider food as contributing to the development of disease is often thought to be unorthodox and alternative.

The critics seem particularly unable to consider that certain foods could produce mental illness. They think schizophrenia is confined to the brain. How, then, could this important and isolated organ be affected by the nutrition of the body? Yet, of course, the brain is entirely dependent on adequate and suitable nutrition.

Remarkably, Dr Carl Pfeiffer has decided to examine the biochemistry of his psychotic patients. He has found high or low levels of nutrients and other body chemicals and, where possible, he has normalised them. He has tested for food sensitivities and blood sugar levels. He has learned about their special problems. He has then grouped his patients into (often overlapping) groups according to symptomatology and devised nutritional therapies for them according to observation and biochemical profile.

So few psychiatrists think these days to ask their patients about their physical symptoms. They still too often concentrate on family relationships as being causative or contributory to the appearance of psychiatric symptoms. Long ago, psychiatrists sought the physical symptoms that were at the root of the trouble. They considered the interaction of diet as Dr Pfeiffer does now.

This book offers hope to many and gives information on how patients can begin to improve their health through nutrition and proper medication. Health is something to be greatly desired by the ill and they need to be taught how to help themselves. We do not know how many mentally ill people could be helped by methods described in this book, but it is worth every psychiatric patient finding out if he can use it to improve his health. We need psychiatrists to take up nutrition as part of their weaponry against disease. If they follow Carl Pfeiffer's leads, they will be a good step along the way of helping their patients to get a lot better than they do on drug treatment alone.

Gwynneth Hemmings
Honorary Secretary
Schizophrenia Association of Great Britain

Part 3

MENTAL ILLNESS
Not all in the mind

One of the greatest shortcomings of human logic is the unquestioned belief that psychological problems, be it of behaviour or intelligence, are influenced only by psychological factors and that physiological problems are influenced only by physiological factors. This presupposes that mind and body are separate, that the energy of mind and of body are two different things. Our experience contradicts this. Alcohol alters your state of mind. Psychological stress makes muscles tense. Ask a chemist, an anatomist and a psychologist to define where the mind starts and the body ends and they will find that the two are intimately interconnected.

11

UNDERSTANDING MENTAL ILLNESS

Before discussing in this book certain factors which relate to mental illness, it is important to understand what we mean by this term. It is often used by layman and specialist alike as an identity tag with no apparent clear–cut definition or understanding.

Defining Mental Illness

In fact, the UK Mental Health Act of 1983 contains no definition. Instead it states, *"In practice the decision as to whether a person is mentally ill is a clinical one and the expression invariably has to be defined by reference to what the doctor says it means in a particular case rather than to any precise legal criteria."*

Blacks Medical Dictionary defines it as, *"problems of feeling, thinking and behaving may be regarded as a mental illness if they become excessive for the particular individual in relation to the difficulties experienced."*

What we commonly understand by the term ' mental illness' is a state of being that falls short of what we consider normal or acceptable. We have all experienced some degree of this. We become unhappy for no apparent reason, or find ourselves reacting explosively to the smallest of stimuli. We hear voices which just won't go away, or feel that we can't go on any more.

In practice, what tends to happen is that a person who continuously suffers from less than normal mental states is labelled depressed, manic–depressive, schizophrenic or with some other mental disorder. He may then carry this label for life, and be tagged as a less than normal human being. Such labels do nothing of actual benefit for the individual, so in defining what we mean by mental illness it is important to avoid a labelling which in itself could contribute to the individual's mental turmoil.

It might therefore be more useful to define our terms in reference to the concept of mental health. If a good state of mental health refers to a condition of feeling stable and satisfied that one is coping adequately with the problems of day to day living, then a mental health problem would refer to a condition where one is NOT coping, where a person is unhappy a lot of the time, frequently feels distressed and is unnaturally and frequently afraid.

With that in mind, for the purposes of this book we will refer to mental illness as being a state of mind in which one is unable to cope with some aspect of life to the point where one's ability to lead a fulfilling life is seriously impaired.

Mind over Matter

Every thought and feeling we have can alter, and is altered by, the chemistry of our body. The mind and body are completely interconnected. One does not exist without the other. The Western concept that we are our minds (I think therefore I am) and that our body is a machine has created this false idea of separation. This false idea generated the notion that mental illness is a result of that part of the machine responsible for mentation, the brain, going wrong. This led to lobotomies and electroconvulsive shock treatment, both of which damage the brain. The other avenue that emerged from this concept of separation was psychoanalysis, that mental illness was the result of problems in the abstract mind, not the physical brain.

Eastern traditions generally work with a different approach to mind and body. They see who we are as the soul, or 'subtle body'. In a different realm, the realm of thought and feelings, manifests our 'astral body'. In the physical realm there exists a 'physical body'. All three co-exist in a human being, each affecting each other. I have found this concept to be helpful in understanding mental health.

Who Suffers?

Mental health problems are as common as heart disease, three times more common than cancer and five times more common than mental handicap. Official figures suggest that 6 million people are sufferers at any one point in time [1]. In the course of a year 12 million adults attending GP surgeries have symptoms of mental illness. Between 1985 and 1990 the number of children up to the age of 14 seen by psychiatric services has approximately doubled 2. In fact out of 100 people that you know up to 20 will be affected at any point in time. Whilst 6 out of 10 people with mental health problems will be formally identified and receiving treatment, an estimated 4 out of 10 are not receiving the help that they need.

As unwelcome as the thought may be, any one of us is a potential sufferer of a mental health problem. We are all subject to a greater or lesser degree to the stresses and strains of daily life, which, for many people may be in addition to a much deeper source of stress or unhappiness coming from a particularly difficult past or present experience. The vast majority (80%) of disorders appear in the form of either anxiety states, depression or stress–related disorders with the remaining 20% being made up of alcohol and drug dependency, dementia, personality and psychotic disorders such as schizophrenia1.

With more than 4 in 10 mentally ill people being considered seriously at risk and therefore in need of specialist treatment, the cost of caring for sufferers is vast. Despite the fact that the numbers of long–stay hospital patients halved during the 1980s, more people are occupying beds for shorter periods or are using out–patient services. In 1991 the official cost of treating those with mental health problems was £3.15 billion -9% of the total NHS expenditure 3. However, many other costs are also incurred, with industry losing £6.2 billion and sickness and invalidity benefit costing a further £1.14 billion a year. None of these figures take into account the cost of informal care taking place in the home, estimated at £1.16 billion and complicated by the fact that 76% of those looked after suffer from physical health problems in addition to mental problems. The total cost to the nation of mental illness exceeds £10 billion, or approximately £200 per person per year 4.

The effects of social deprivation on mental health cannot be disputed. Suicide rates are 11 times higher among the unemployed and 53 people per thousand are being admitted to psychiatric hospitals from deprived areas as opposed to 19 per thousand as a national average 5. However, this still begs the question as to why some people seem to cope reasonably well with a given situation while others will start to manifest the symptoms of mental illness. The answer to this is, of course, not cut and dried, but an increasing body of evidence points to one of the underlying causes of mental health problems being an actual physical or chemical imbalance in the body.

Getting the Right Diagnosis

A study by a Stanford University California Professor of Law and Psychology, Dr Rosenhan clearly demonstrates this problem5. The study proved, basically that insanity can easily be faked in front of professionals who do not use objective diagnostic tools such as psychometric assessments and biochemical tests.

Dr Rosenhan and seven others, including three psychologists, and a psychiatrist, gained admission to twelve hospitals on the East and West Coasts of the USA by faking mental illness (eleven of the hospitals were totally funded by public money). The story they told to gain admission was that they 'heard voices'. Asked what the voices said he replied that they were often unclear but as far as he could tell they said 'empty', 'hollow' and 'thud'. However, once admitted to the hospital, they acted in a normal manner. In therapy, they answered all questions truthfully, including those about their childhood and their current areas of interest. They engaged in normal activities in the hospitals and, short of revealing their true purpose, they did everything possible to gain their release. Yet only the other patients in the hospitals were able to tell that these 'pseudopatients' were sane. The first three pseudopatients to be hospitalised took careful notes. Their accurate accounts show that 35 of a total of 118 regular patients were suspicious of them. Referring to their continual note-taking, one regular patient remarked: "You're not crazy. You're a journalist or a professor. You're checking up on the hospital."

The hospital staff, however, were not able to detect the pseudopatients' sanity. One nurse saw the note-taking as a symptom of a sick compulsion: "Engages in writing behaviour," she put on the patient's chart. This led Dr Rosenhan to conclude that, "once a patient is designated as abnormal, all his other behaviours and characteristics are coloured by that label." Whether this generalisation is true or not, the inability of the hospitals to diagnose properly, or even suspect something, shows how the thin line between sanity and insanity may be blurred. Proper use of the medical model entails careful differential diagnosis, which draws this line firmly in view for both the staff and patient.

None of the pseudopatients were discharged as cured; all bore the label 'schizophrenia in remission'. In other words, it would seem they were still 'insane'. With the 'schizophrenia' on their record, they would have to bear this stigma, and even be expected to behave as a schizophrenic again, concludes Dr. Rosenhan.

The single uniform and simple disperception which the pseudopatients reported in their first interview at the hospitals was the only evidence of 'schizophrenia' - that waste basket diagnosis. Psychiatrists can be so trusting as to assume that reasons do not occur for anyone to actually want to report a disperception unless so afflicted. The error of course is the lack of follow-up with objective tests, which were never given to the patients! On a test such a the EWI (Experiential World Inventory, a diagnostic test), the patient can report disperceptions in a setting where he has no fear of recrimination, in a more or less objective fashion. There is no possibility that 200 answers can be faked. The point is that there is no reason to report disperceptions unless they are real (ie. the walls look curved, I hear voices that aren't there, etc.). Anyone who wilfully fakes answers on this kind of test is, literally, out of his mind.

One observation that Dr Rosenhan made, as a result of this study, was that mental illness carries with it a connotation entirely different from that of a physical disorder. The Diagnostic and Statistical Manual of the American Psychiatric Association, the official bible of psychiatric diagnoses, might have one believe that the sane are always clearly distinguished from the insane, and that 'schizophrenia' (waste basket) is always treated as objectively and straightforwardly as a broken leg. Rosenhan found that, in actual practice, this was not the case. For example, sensible questions asked by the pseudopatients were frequently ignored. One patient stopped a doctor and asked: "Excuse me, Dr.........., could you tell me when I am eligible for grounds privileges?" The doctor replied: "Good morning, Dave. How are you today?" and moved on without waiting for an answer or answering the patient's question. Not only was the credibility of the patients impaired in this way (presumably because of their diagnostic labels), but they were denied privacy even in matters of personal hygiene. They reported feeling depersonalised, even though they knew they did not belong in the mental hospital.

Doctors Diagnose 21% of Sick Patients as Imposters!

Dr Rosenhan further wondered whether the atrocious diagnostic performance of the hospital staffs merely reflected their professional caution. Having once been informed that a patient was hearing voices, perhaps the psychiatrists felt obliged to alert all future doctors to the possibility of trouble. Thus, Rosenhan wondered if his findings resulted from the greater inclination of physicians to call a healthy person sick than sick person healthy. To check on this, he provided an esteemed psychiatric hospital, one of those involved in his first study, with yet another opportunity to redeem their reputation for adequate and proper diagnosis. The staff was informed that at some time during the next three months, one or more pseudopatients would once again attempt to be admitted into their hospital. The staff members were asked to rate each person who presented himself for admission as to the likelihood that the patient was a pseudopatient. Of the succeeding 193 patients admitted, 41 (or 21%) of them were judged, with a high degree of confidence, to be pseudopatients by at least one member of staff. The joke, again, was on the hospital staff. No pseudopatients at all had been sent to the hospital!

We can conclude that:

1 psychiatric diagnosis, without objective laboratory tests and psychometric tests, are frequently in error and useless
2 lacking an accurate diagnostic method a label should not be applied, and
3 a fresh approach to psychiatric diagnosis and care is needed.

What Divides Abnormal Behaviour from Mental Illness?

A valid point for debate is whether certain abnormal behaviour qualifies as mental illness. Patients who have certain mental symptoms after strokes or infections of the brain present no problem in being considered ill. In contrast, there is a group of disorders listed, in the standard nomenclature of the American Psychiatric Association, as 'character and behaviour disorders'. There is nothing in these terms to suggest any organic or physiological derangement, so to call them mental illness, although currently fashionable, is stretching the term considerably.

Manic-Depression

Somewhere between these extremes are patients with two major psychoses: the schizophrenias and manic-depressive psychosis. It has become popular also to regard manic-depressive psychosis as 'better' than schizophrenia. Manic-depressive psychosis has long been felt to have a biochemical basis, and anyway, doctors claim 'it is only a disorder of emotions, the patient isn't really crazy'. Perhaps this is, in part, because intellectual functioning may be less impaired than in one of the severe schizophrenias.

Schizophrenia has become a dirty word, a diagnosis to be whispered, and often to be concealed from patient, family, or friends. Again, a broken leg or even blindness would be more bearable, because it is visible, explicable, and being plainly physical, is something one can live with. Socially determined bias has a role in the way the two kinds of major mental disease are regarded. In a way, to be depressed is noble. Kings and even Abraham Lincoln had spells of depression. 'To be good you must suffer' is stated in many religions.

Yet the schizophrenias, about which some people have such strong and irrational feelings (no doubt because of their own fears or other emotional reactions), strike everywhere throughout all of mankind. The commonly quoted figure of 1% of all humanity is probably far short of the actual incidence. We should add to this estimate the walking wounded who are never seen by any doctor, since only one-third of those afflicted need be hospitalised. We must also add the teenager who commits suicide before an accurate diagnosis is made. Thus the problem is one which is important from the viewpoint of numbers, as well as individual misery. Heart disease may cause more deaths, but the schizophrenias cause more heart-ache. Given a choice, most of us who have tasted adult freedom would prefer a quick death rather than the aimless custody of any mental institution, which may be the fate of the untreated schizophrenic.

Understanding Schizophrenia

There are many conflicting descriptions and explanations for the schizophrenias, but at a basic level, there is usually little difficulty in making a preliminary diagnosis; and there is usually agreement among doctors in making the diagnosis, even though they may disagree about the possible causes and the ultimate outcome for any given patient. Since the schizophrenias may vary from simple (but abnormal) feelings of disperception or persecution to complete loss of contact with reality, the doctor hesitates to apply the term schizophrenia to the mild forms of disorder. Instead he uses the terms 'schizoid personality', 'schizophrenic reaction', or other such words. The doctor really means 'I am puzzled and will sit on the fence until I see what happens to you in the next year or so as you free wheel through life with or without medication'.

Uniform features of the schizophrenias on which doctors agree, are that disorders of thought, perception and experience or interaction occur. The schizophrenias are a subjective or personal mental aberration, with no clear or reliable external manifestations. A broken bone would be easier to bear, because it is objective and obviously real. The lack of firm, objective signs is perhaps the crux of the continuing argument as to whether the schizophrenias may have any physiological or biochemical basis.

Some of the schizophrenias can be likened to a nightmare state from which there is no certain awakening. Even more accurately, the experiences of schizophrenics are reproduced in certain toxic or feverous states. The normal person on recovery from a high fever with delusions, can breathe a great sigh of relief at the thought that his experience was temporary and will not occur again. The person under the influence of the hallucinogenic drug LSD has the clock as his best friend, since the drug-induced schizophrenia will wear off with time. For the person with the worst kind of the schizophrenias, however, the abnormal state has no let up and may be a continuing nightmare.

Understanding Paranoia

What brings the patient and doctor together? The things which characterise the untreated schizophrenias can be separated into classes: those which bother the patient and those which bother those around the patient. The two botherations may not be the same. In fact, there is often considerable friction between the patient and others. Consider the case of the man who says he has visions and hears the voice of Jesus. Hallucinations are considered by doctors to be evidence of psychosis; but what if this man is a lay preacher to one of the churches which teach that if you only have enough faith. Christ will appear in person? To him then, the people who say he is mentally ill are merely a bunch of non-believers. The preacher is an example of the fact that leadership and secondary gain frequently go with the delusions and hallucinations of many paranoids. Many of the stresses and frustrations of everyday life could be assuaged if one had a firm belief in being a chosen child or disciple of God (many people have this without being delusional about it, of course).

This discord creates certain practical difficulties. Consider the case of a paranoid young woman. She keeps insisting to her family that she is carrying the new Christ-child in her abdomen because she hasn't had a menstrual period for three months. This lack of a menstrual period is usually owing to a lack of zinc in her body because of stress and eating a zinc deficient diet high in refined sugar. The family is upset and annoyed by her continued delusion as well as by her untidiness, lack of co-operation and general unpleasantness around the house. Complaints are then made to the family doctor, but by the family, not by the patient. The patient refuses flatly to even talk to the doctor, insisting that she is in good health: 'It's just that my family don't understand me and my new role in society.' This kind of situation can create a dilemma for the doctor. Although the diagnosis is reasonably clear, should the doctor insist on treating a patient who has not asked for help? Of course, if the patient asks for treatment there is no problem. If the patient presents some clear evidence that he or she may harm someone, intervention is clearly justified. However, aside from the unethical taint of unsolicited treatment, a major goal is to keep patients out of the hospitals whenever possible. Sometimes that alone is a victory, because with some of our present mental hospitals, there is the probability that the patient may be better off at home. One situation that creates great difficulty occurs when the doctor suspects that the patient may be suicidal or homicidal. Since the conservation of human life has high priority, the physician must try to treat the patient. Being only human and acting on the basis of insufficient tests, the doctor is sometimes wrong, no matter how great his ability. Patients, after such a false alarm, are often bitter and unforgiving. Indeed, they frequently incorporate the memory of such a forced hospitalisation into their delusional systems.

12

THE NUTRITION CONNECTION

Quantum leaps in our understanding about how thoughts and feelings become disordered have been made in the last 50 years. The mysteries of the human brain are being unravelled as we identify the functions of different aspects of the brain, and how brain cells, called neurons , communicate with each other with electrical and chemical messages. The chemical messengers are called neurotransmitters and it is well established that imbalances in these neurotransmitters can result in depression, hallucinations, anxiety, insomnia, blank mind, learning difficulties, poor impulse control and other mental health problems.

While some mental health problems may have little to do with the 'hardware', instead requiring support and guidance from friends and counsellors, there is little doubt that many people with mental health problems do have real chemical imbalances that predispose them to becoming depressed, anxious or confused.

Until recently the only available method of helping to balance the chemistry of the brain was through a variety of drugs which tend to dampen emotional and mental activity, and, in many cases, have undesirable side-effects including addiction. Only when scientists started to examine what the brain and nervous system was actually made of did the importance of nutrition, the food you eat, become apparent.

The brain is made entirely out of food molecules. It concentrates large amounts of complex essential fats, vitamins, minerals, proteins and other nutrients. No less than sixty per cent of all nutrients passed from the mother to the developing infant during pregnancy are used by the brain for its development. Even in a fully grown adult up to thirty per cent of all energy derived from food is used by the brain. Human beings have a brain that is ten times heavier in relation to body weight than almost every other animal and, we have learnt, are totally dependent on a diet rich in nutrients for mental and emotional health.

With these discoveries medical researchers started to investigate whether some mental health problems could be corrected by giving certain nutrients. This approach was called 'orthomolecular medicine' meaning medicine that gives the body the right (ortho) molecules to maintain health. Two psychiatrists in Canada, Dr Abram Hoffer and Dr Humphrey Osmond, started to report amazing recoveries in patients labelled as schizophrenic using large amounts of vitamins and minerals. An American doctor and biochemist, Dr Carl Pfeiffer, identified types of mental illness that could be corrected by specific diets and nutrients. He identified zinc deficiency as a cause of mental illness and developed nutritional approaches for correcting neurotransmitter imbalances. He believed that, if there was a drug that could affect mental health, then the right nutrients could achieve the same result, or better, without the side effects.

The Four Pillars of Mental Health

Since the pioneering research of the 1960's nutrition has been identified as a major factor in hyperactivity, learning difficulties, delinquent behaviour, depression, anxiety, schizophrenia, insomnia, memory loss, anorexia - in fact almost every known type of mental health problem has been positively helped by nutritional therapy.

Nutritional deficiencies are not simply the result of eating a bad diet. Modern man is exposed to many chemicals which interfere with how the nutrients from food work. These are called 'anti-nutrients' and include certain kinds of food additives, household chemicals, drugs and inhaled pollutants from smoking, exhaust and industrial pollution. For example, lead in petrol and cadmium in cigarettes are two 'anti-nutrients' that accumulate in the brain and affect behaviour and mood. Since the 1940's over 6,500 totally new, man-made chemicals have been introduced into our food and homes.

The consequence of taking in too little beneficial nutrients and too many harmful anti-nutrients can easily affect the level and balance of both physical and mental energy. Without sufficient energy it is hard to concentrate and hard to cope with the stresses and demands of modern

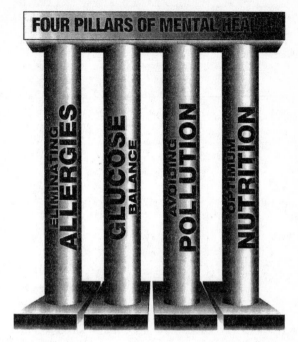

Figure 12: The Four Pillars

living. This often leads to the overconsumption of 'stimulants' such as sugar, tea, coffee, cigarettes, chocolate and stimulant drugs in an attempt to boost energy. However, in the long run, stimulants deplete energy, as well as predisposing the user to states of anxiety and hyperactivity. The overconsumption of stimulants is therefore another contributory factor that leads to mental and emotional imbalance. Conversely, over-stimulation as experienced in states of anxiety, may lead to the use of 'depressants' including alcohol and tranquilliser drugs.

As well as identifying the role of nutrients, anti-nutrients, stimulants and depressants in mental health research over the past 30 years has proven the very real existence of food allergies or intolerances that result in mental and emotional symptoms.

The combination of any of the following: sub-optimum nutrition, exposure to anti-nutrients, over-use of sugar, stimulants and

NEUROTRANSMITTER:	ACETYLCHOLINE		HISTAMINE	
	Excess	Deficiency	Excess	Deficiency
Signs and Symptoms	Excessive vigilance & movement Seizures Asthma Increased dreaming Excess salivation	Memory deficit Flaccidity Decreased dreaming Dry mouth	Obsessions Compulsions Energetic High libido Allergies Migraines Needs little sleep Drug resistant	Paranoia Lethargy Overweight Reacts to drugs Hallucinations Excessive need for sleep High pain threshold
Precursor Amino Acid:	Serine, choline		Histidine	
Co-factor Nutrients:	Pantothenic acid, choline, DMAE, pyroglutamate, manganese		Vitamin B6, copper, zinc, manganese	
Inhibitory factors:	Several drugs		Copper, alcohol, certain drugs (anti-histamines), heavy metals	

depressants, and food allergies or intolerances - is now thought to be a very real contributor to mental and emotional health problems. The correction of these factors often results in substantial improvement.

Psychoanalysis or Neuroanalysis?

Advances in biotechnology are unravelling the mysteries of the mind. Now, the chemical neurotransmitters required for all thought and memory processes can actually be measured. Some scientists believe that balance of these neurotransmitters help to determine our mental and emotional characteristics. Neurotransmitter imbalances may also be the underlying cause of some kinds of mental illness and schizophrenia. Orthomolecular psychiatry, in which individuals are given the right (ortho) nutrients to correct brain chemistry disorders, in preference to drugs, is breaking new ground and promising rich rewards in the field of psychiatry and mental health.

That neurotransmitters, chemicals that allow messages to pass from neuron to neuron, are essential for brain function is nothing new. In fact, modern day neuro-psychiatry is based on this premise. Most

ADRENALINE		DOPAMINE		SEROTONIN	
Excess	Deficiency	Excess	Deficiency	Excess	Deficiency
Insomnia	Narcolepsy	Sexual	Sexual	Narcolepsy	Insomnia
Mania	Depression	arousal	disinterest		Anxiety
Hypertension	Hypotension	Psychosis	Agitation		Impulsive
Migraine	Stimulant craving		Parkinson's disease		behaviour
Tyrosine, phenylalanine		Tyrosine, phenylalanine		Tryptophan	
Vitamin B3, B6, C, folic acid, copper, magnesium		Vitamin B6, biotin, iron		Vitamin B3, B6, iron	
Excess use of stimulants		Several drugs		Oestrogen, heavy metals	

Adapted from Jaffe, Kruesi, Int Clin Nut Rev, 12, 1, p 9-26 1992

drugs are thought to work precisely because they encourage or block the action of specific neurotransmitters. Yet, few patients prescribed powerful drugs that alter brain chemistry are ever tested for neurotransmitter levels. In the not too distant future they may be because tests already exist to determine whether excesses or deficiencies of key neurotransmitters exist.

Such tests are allowing for a radical reclassification of mental health problems based on concrete biological data rather than subjective assessment. Symptom patterns are beginning to emerge alongside the new 'neuro-data'. For example, poor memory, infrequent dreams, lethargy and poor saliva production are associated with acetylcholine deficiency. Compulsive, obsessive and hyperactive behaviour, migraines and a high sex drive are associated with histamine excess. Insomnia, anxiety and impulsive behaviour may be the result of a serotonin deficiency. Imbalances in other neurotransmitters such as adrenalin, dopamine, glutamine and GABA may underlie tendencies to insomnia, depression, mania, schizophrenia, seizures, Parkinson's and other common mental health problems (see table above).

These tests, as yet unavailable in the UK, may form the basis of a more accurate diagnosis of mental health problems in the years to come. But orthomolecular psychiatry isn't just changing the diagnostic procedures, its stimulating a move away from psychotropic drugs, towards the use of nutrients to bring brain biochemistry back in balance. This is because the precursor materials that allow neurotransmitters to be formed are principally amino acids, constituents of protein supplied from the diet. The enzymes required for the formation of neurotransmitters depend upon co-factors, principally vitamins and minerals. By altering a person's nutrient intake neurotransmitter imbalances can often be corrected. For example, a lack of adrenalin is one cause for depression and narcolepsy, excessive sleeping and sleepiness. Adrenalin is formed from the amino acid tyrosine. Co-factors are copper, magnesium, vitamin C, B3, B6 and folic acid. The orthomolecular approach involves supplying these nutrients, rather than psychotropic drugs - working with the design of the human body rather than against it. Spectacular results have been achieved using this approach, although nutrients do take longer to act than most drugs.

Psycho-Immunity

Why do neurotransmitter imbalances develop? This key question is difficult to research since it requires long-term studies 'tracking' people without imbalances and seeing which factors are associated with developing imbalances and the onset of mental illness. Such studies have yet to be performed. The likely origin involves a combination of an inherited tendency to certain imbalances, brought out by inappropriate nutrition. The question becomes even more complex when you consider that inherited tendencies may themselves be the result of inappropriate nutrition in the mother, especially during pregnancy. Other factors include exposure to 'anti-nutrients' such as heavy metals, and immune system abnormalities. Dr Russell Jaffe, formerly of the Princeton Bio Center estimates that 15% of the schizophrenic patients they see are 'immunoreactive' meaning that they have developed food and chemical sensitivities. In the long-term this can exacerbate nutrient deficiencies and disrupt normal metabolism of amino acids, carbohydrates and fats, thereby influencing neurotransmitter balance.

Causes of Schizophrenia

A significant proportion of so-called schizophrenics fall into one or more of five clinical types 1. These are: the low histamine 'histapenic' type; the high histamine 'histadelic' type; the 'pyroluric' type; the nutrient deficient 'co-factor depleted' type; and the 'immunoreactive' type. These different types often overlap and are each explained in the chapters that follow.

But can schizophrenias really be defined as simply as that? Can life or individuals be categorised that easily? No, indeed! The fact is that if we include fevers, environmental pains and drug reactions, there must be a hundred ways to go crazy and be diagnosed as schizophrenic. Our patients realise that we are carefully sorting out the different causes of their craziness and they are usually tolerant of any mistakes since we are doing everything we can to get at the root cause of their illness.

New Frontiers

One of the most important advances in the last twenty years is the increasing understanding of the interaction between the brain and nervous system and the immune system. This field, sometimes called 'psychoneuroimmunology' is as complex as it's name! However, it is becoming increasingly clear that immune reactions, often to foods or chemicals, can have a profound effects on the the brain, and subsequently of mood and behaviour. Immune reactions are more likely to occur in nutrient deficient people, with the use of psychotropic drugs, tobacco, recreational drugs, including alcohol predisposing people to deficiency.

The role of essential fats in brain function is also providing promise for new treatments. Over 20% of the dry weight of the brain is made from essential fatty acids (EFA's). Numerous studies have shown low levels of EFA's in schizophrenics. These EFA's help balance neurotransmitters, so a deficiency can lead to over-excitation. Supplementing EFAs has been shown to help many sufferers 2. Recently, Dr Iain Glen, from the mental health department of Aberdeen University, found that 80% of schizophrenics are EFA deficient. He gave 50 patients EFA supplements and reported a dramatic response 3.

Mental Illness - The Way Forward

With one in a hundred people is diagnosed as suffering from schizophrenia. and many more suffer from depression, anxiety, extreme fears and phobias, help is badly needed. But what treatment is available? For the seriously mentally ill this means psychiatric help. Some psychiatrists view mental illness as a psychologically based disease, a perplexing nightmare often intertwined with suspicious family interactions. The treatment may be endless psychoanalysis and an endless drain on financial resources with little more than a slim chance of help. (As one patient said after years of psychoanalysis, 'I may know myself a lot better but I'm still mentally ill!'). Other psychiatrists lean more heavily on drug treatments, but these too have only a small chance of really helping. Many psychotherapeutic drugs leave the patient drowsy and 'drugged' and have nasty side-effects (for which other drugs have to be given) as well as carrying the risk of brain damage. There was no alternative until recently!

Part 4

MENTAL ILLNESS
The modern approach

The current approach to mental health problems mainly involves drug therapy or psychotherapy, neither of which have an impressive success rate. We believe, and present the evidence in this book, that a significant proportion of mentally unwell people do not need drugs nor respond well to psychotherapy. This is because the primary cause of their problem may neither be a lack of drugs, nor a lack of psychological insight or support, but a chemical imbalance that affects how they think and feel brought on by years of poor nutrition and exposure to environmental toxins.

After 30 years of positive research we believe that the time has come for another option, nutrition counselling, to be made widely available to those with mental health problems.

13

THE MODERN CLASSIFICATION OF MENTAL HEALTH PROBLEMS

There are many ways to develop mental health problems and many factors, physical, biochemical and psychological, before imprisoning people in the strait-jacket of long term drug therapy. Listed below are a number of possible causes for mental illness and disperceptions that cause schizophrenia.

The modern approach to mental illness involves keeping an open mind to all these possible contributory causes, understanding that, in most cases, more than one apply. Diagnoses are made on the basis of objective biochemical tests and subjective symptom assessment. Once symptoms are gone and test results are normalised the patient can be declared better. Dr Abram Hoffer, a psychiatrist who has pioneered this approach since the 1950's, claims a 90% success rate in acute schizophrenia, with thousands of cases to prove it. His definition of cure is threefold:

1 Free from symptoms
2 Able to socialise with family and community
3 Paying income tax

The chapters which follow explain many of these major types, how to identify them and, most important of all, how nutrition can help correct and prevent them.

Well-known

Dementia paralytic
Porphyria
Drug intoxications
Folic acid/B12 deficiency
Heavy metal toxicity

Pellagra - niacin deficiency
Hypothyroidism
Homocysteinuria
Sleep deprivation

Less well-known

Hypoglycemia
Cerebral allergy
Histapenia -copper excess
Pyroluria
Chronic candida infection
Prostaglandin/EFA deficiency
Serotonin imbalance

Psychomotor epilepsy
Wheat-gluten sensitivity
Histadelia
Wilson's disease
Huntington's chorea
Dopamine excess

Almost unknown

Endorphin imbalance
Prolactin excess
Lysine, histidine imbalance

Serine excess
Dialysis therapy
Interferon, amantadine, anti-
viral drugs, any drug toxicity
Platelets deficient in MHO

14

OVERCOMING DEPRESSION

Liz started suffering from depression at the age of 14. By the time she was 17 she had become extremely anxious, fearful and depressed and was hearing voices. She was put on three drugs - Sulpiride and Depixol injections, plus Kemadrin to offset the side-effects of the other drugs. The drugs somewhat sedated her but she continued to suffer from extreme depression and anxiety and continued to hear voices in her head. She also had psychotherapy but neither this, nor the drugs made any real difference.

She consulted a nutrition counsellor who identified chronic nutritional deficiencies and an excessive level of histamine, an neurotransmitter that affects the brain. Within six months she was no longer depressed, and rarely heard voices or became anxious. She came off all medication and continued to improve. She is now perfectly healthy and happy and recently gave birth to a baby girl. She experienced no post-natal depression.

There are many potential nutrition-related causes of depression including nutrient deficiencies, glucose intolerance and allergy, all of which are discussed in this book. One common contributory cause is an excess of histamine, known as histadelia. This is mostly an inherited trait.

Since histamine speeds up metabolism, providing more heat, and since vitamin C is an anti-histamine, we think that when our ancestors lost the ability to make vitamin C, a fate they share only with guinea pigs, flying bats and other primates, this put them at an advantage in colder climates during and after the Ice Age.

But histamine also causes allergic reactions, increased production of mucus and saliva, a tendency to hyperactivity, compulsive behaviour and depression. Some of these traits can be an advantage, but when histamine levels are not controlled, they can lead to chronic depression and even suicide. Marilyn Monroe, Judy Garland and Shane McNeill, son of Eugene McNeill, are three examples of likely histadelics who died a suicidal death.

The histadelic patient comprises about 20% of so-called schizophrenics and a majority of depressed patients. This estimate is based on the many patients who were treated over the last 30 years. The histadelic person is often the problem patient at psychiatric clinics and hospitals.

Are you Histadelic?

Do you:

1 Sneeze in bright sunlight?
2 Feel you were shy and over-sensitive as a teenager?
3 Cry, salivate and feel nauseous easily?
4 Hear your pulse in your head on the pillow at night?
5 Get referred itches when you scratch your leg?
6 Have frequent back aches, stomach aches, muscle cramps?
7 Have easy orgasm with sex?
8 Have regular headaches and seasonal allergies?
9 Have inner tension and occasional depression?
10 Have abnormal fears, compulsions, rituals?
11 Think you are a light sleeper?
12 Burn up foods rapidly?
13 Sometimes have suicidal thoughts?
14 Tolerate a lot of alcohol and other 'downers'?
15 Have little body hair and lean build?
16 Have large ears and long fingers and toes?
17 Belong to an all boy family?

If a majority of the above apply you may benefit from:
- A low-protein, high complex carbohydrate diet
- Calcium 500mg, am and pm with
- Methionine, 500mg, am and pm
- plus a basic supplement programme (see page 198)
- But you should avoid folic acid and multivitamins which contain folic acid because these can raise histamine levels.

Our first contact with histadelia occurred in a biochemical and psychiatric study of out-patient schizophrenics. Two out of nine chronic patients on whom we had extensive data and repeated visits showed significant positive correlations between blood histamine and the Experimental World Inventory (EWI), a psychological measure of stability. In other words, both the highly-elevated EWI score and the blood histamine decreased as the patient got better.

Histadelia usually runs in families, with the onset at around 20 years of age. The easily elicited history of suicide, depression and allergies among near and distant relatives is a strong indication of possible histadelia. This disorder has probably been termed familial psychotic depression in the past. The undiagnosed histadelic patient is treated as a schizophrenic but the patient does not respond to any of the usual drug therapies,electroshock or insulin coma therapy. We have now treated over a thousand of these patients and our experience provides many important signs that help in making early diagnosis.

Histadelics are Compulsive People

Disperceptions, obsessions, compulsions, thought disorder, blank mind, abnormal fears, constant suicidal depression, easy crying,confusion and blank mind may all occur. The symptom of blank mind is elicited by asking if the patient can visualise the face of her mother or visualise why, on a motorway, she might be directed to turn left though she actually wants to turn right on to a new motorway (clover leaf turn). She often cannot visualise these things.

These people are fast oxidisers and may have drug, alcohol and sugar addiction. Histamine furthers rapid oxidation of foodstuffs so the histadelic patient may be the thin individual with the hollow leg: 'I can eat or drink anything without gaining weight'.

Metabolic Symptoms

Because of the high histamine level the histadelic can cry at the slightest provocation. Histamine produces a good flow of saliva so the teeth are frequently free of cavities. The metabolic rate is high so the patient has minimal fat - an attractive body figure is the result. Since Marilyn Monroe was probably histadelic we can, at this late date, understand better her remark to news photographers, 'You always take pictures of my body but my most perfect feature is my teeth - I have no cavities.' With good salivary flow teeth are well bathed in saliva and the histadelic may have the habit of wiping saliva from the corners of the mouth with thumb and index finger. Like a drug addict, he may be hooked on excess sugar in coffee or tea. A history of allergies or periodic headache and sensitivity to pain is also common. When blood is taken or an injection of B12 is given, the patient may cry out or squirm because he has a very low pain threshold. Patients will not have excessive body or extremity hair. In men the beard is usually light and there are few chest hairs. The natural hair colour is usually brunette or black. Histadelics usually have relatively long fingers and toes, with the second toe being longer than the big toe. When Marilyn Monroe met her sister Berniece for the first time, at the age of 25, Berniece says in an interview "the most exciting thing was discovering our toes. See how the second toe is longer than the rest. Marilyn had the same thing." Their mother, Gladys, spent many years in a mental institution, diagnosed as a schizophrenic.

The histadelic usually has an easy and well sustained orgasm and therefore the label of nymphomania may occasionally be applied. We have also seen some depressed children with high blood histamine but these children frequently have lead poisoning which also raises blood histamine. Histadelic patients have the most severe insomnia of any subdivision of the 'schizophrenias'. In severe cases doses of five 100mg pentobarbital tablets are often needed at bedtime, along with chlorpromazine to get a good night's sleep. One such patient living alone swallowed and slept through a dose of twenty-seven pentobarbital capsules! Ordinarily, we medics worry about ten being swallowed at a single dose.

Drugs Don't Help

These overtreated and mistreated patients have frequently made the rounds of the best psychiatric hospitals where large doses of chlorpromazine or fluphenazine are often ineffective. Electroshock does little and insulin coma therapy is useless. The patient on 10mg fluphenazine may seem like a wooden statue because of the drug-induced muscle effects - and the psychiatrist may now say catatonia has set in! This catatonia, of course, responds to a decrease in the fluphenazine dosage or the daily use of Cogentin - an antidote to the muscle contractions. The anti-depressant drugs such as amitriptyline or MAO inhibitors (Parstelin or Nardil) are ineffective. Lithium in a low dose of 600-900mg per day is somewhat effective; larger doses are not more effective. L-tryptophan in the usual dose of 1g at bedtime may produce a prolonged two to three hour blushing sensation and cardiovascular reaction, apparently because of the histadelic's rapid conversion of tryptophan to the brain chemical, serotonin.

Vitamins C and B3 Don't Help Either

Nor do these people respond to the classical meganutrient (B3, vitamin C) therapy first used by Drs Hoffer and Osmond. If the B vitamin, folic acid, is given, the patient definitely gets worse. B12 injection is tolerated, however, and may moderate depression.

What does work is calcium supplementation, which releases some of the body's stores of histamine, and the natural amino acid methionine, which helps to detoxify histamine by methylation - the usual mode of detoxification of histamine in the human body. Phenytoin, the anti-epilepsy drug (trade marked Dilantin in the USA) is also an anti-folic acid drug. Phenytoin in a dose of 100mg, am and pm will usually provide some relief for the severely depressed or compulsive patient. However, the methionine plus calcium combined with zinc and manganese is often sufficient so we can sometimes omit the use of phenytoin. The same regime of zinc, manganese, calcium, methionine (and phenytoin) provides successful treatment in many severely allergic patients who are not depressed. The most effective diet may be one that is low in protein with adequate vegetables and fruit.

Testing for Histamine

Specialised laboratories can actually test histamine levels in the blood (see Useful Addresses on page 200) which is the best way of determining your histamine status.

As with all chronic depressives, the prognosis in histadelia must be cautiously guarded. Patients may stop their nutritional programme, become suicidal, and the grim reaper may win. In general, if the patient stays with the nutritional programme, the depressions and compulsions are kept in check. For example, we started treating one young man for histadelia ten years ago. He had been in mental hospitals from the age of 17 until he was 26. However, he has not been hospitalised since our treatment commenced and is now a productive citizen. While depression is often lifted early on, compulsions with abnormal fears are the most difficult to treat and are also the last symptom to go.

Drug Addicts are Histadelic

Having tested 12 hard-core drug addicts and found them all to be high in histamine, we voice the strong opinion that more can be done to correct biochemical imbalance in the drug addict. We know that heroin and methadone are both strong histamine releasing agents. The histadelic person is depressed, compulsive and has abnormal thinking. Therefore heroin, methadone, uppers, downers, alcohol and sugar are often craved to compensate for these feelings. The compulsive day-in-day-out drinker of alcohol is usually found to be histadelic. Moderation must be taught tactfully to these individuals as they slowly but surely improve on nutrition.

The Threat of Suicide

The greatest problem in the severely depressed histadelic is the constant threat of suicide. An understanding relative or spouse living with the patient is the best safeguard. Character disorder, as in the drug addict, is always a problem and the remembrance of how high and powerful the patient felt on drugs is a problem. We can never meet this degree of mental over-alertness with good nutrition. We can make the patient feel normal but not hypomanic. For some of these compulsive patients normality is just not enough.

15

CONQUERING FEARS, PHOBIAS AND HALLUCINATIONS

Histamine is an important brain chemical and is involved in all sorts of reactions, including those to pain and allergies, causing tears to flow, excessive mucus, saliva and other bodily secretions. While too much can be a cause of mental health problems, from a careful study of the data from thousands of schizophrenic patients, we found that 50 per cent have a low blood level of histamine which rises to normal levels as they improve. This is called histapenia.

What Causes low Histamine?

The histapenic patient is not only low in histamine but is also often loaded with copper. Thus, both histamine depletion and copper excess may produce behavioural abnormalities. Instead of blaming the family, or the 'schizophrenic mother' who is accused of loving her offspring too much or too little, the finding of high copper in a patient's blood shifts the blame to the environment - usually to the copperized drinking water resulting from the use of copper in water pipes. The concept grows that some metals now called trace elements or micronutrients, such as zinc and manganese, may be deficient, or copper may be in excess, in some types of 'schizophrenias'.

The low histamine or histapenic person also has some distinctive characteristics, as shown on the next page. These are most pronounced in histapenic schizophrenics, but they exist in a diminished form in a large proportion of the general population.

While the patient who is high in histamine may have depression, obsession and suicide, disperception and thought disorder, histapenic

Are you histapenic?

Do you have any of these characteristics?

1 Canker sores
2 Difficult orgasm with sex
3 No headaches or allergies
4 Heavy growth of body hair
5 Excess fat in lower extremities
6 Many dental fillings
7 Ideas of grandeur
8 Undue suspicion of people
9 The feeling that someone controls your mind
10 Seeing or hearing things abnormally
11 The ability to stand pain well
12 Ringing in the ears

If a majority of the above apply you may benefit from:
• Niacin 500mg, am and pm (will cause a blushing sensation)
• Folic acid, 1000mcg each am
• B12 injection, weekly or daily supplementation
• L-Tryptophan, 1,000mg at bedtime
• Zinc and manganese daily
• High-protein diet
• plus a basic supplement programme (see page 198)

patients have all the classic symptoms of 'schizophrenia', including anxiety, paranoia and hallucinations.

Schizophrenics may have low levels of zinc and manganese and high levels of copper, iron, mercury or lead. The last two are, of course, poisons, but the poisoning may produce symptoms which mimic those of 'schizophrenia'. This has been well documented for mercury and lead.

The Copper Controversy

One of the earliest studies implicating high copper in schizophrenia was carried out in 1941 by Dr Heilmeyer and colleagues. They reported findings of elevated serum copper levels in 23 out of 37 schizophrenics. In subsequent studies the same authors found similar serum copper elevation in some manic depressives and epileptics, and also in some cases of alcohol intoxication, infectious disease and cancer. Modern analytic techniques have since confirmed the frequent prevalence of high copper individuals suffering from these disorders.

These original findings did stimulate some interest in copper research in schizophrenia on the details of high copper were essentially verified by several workers in the subsequent years [1]. Brenner made an extensive study of the serum copper levels in childhood 'schizophrenia' under different physiological and pathological conditions. In children with definite schizophrenic symptoms, he found extremely high serum copper levels, in contrast to the findings for children with mental retardation and other brain disorders. Brenner also found that more than a third of adult schizophrenics had high copper levels, which were not detectable during periods of spontaneous remission. But not all researchers have had such positive results [2].

A very careful and well-controlled study on copper metabolism in 122 schizophrenics was performed by Ozek in 1957 [3]. No less than two-thirds of patients had high copper levels, especially among those described as having an 'acute' condition. (No difference in the red blood cell levels of copper or ceruloplasmin levels was detected. Ceruloplasmin is the copper containing serum protein which contains the enzyme, serum oxidase.)

In 1957, Dr. Ackerfeldt reported elevated levels of the copper-based enzyme, serum oxidase, in adult schizophrenics. He was the first to make this observation. This was then confirmed in a study of 250 schizophrenics which also found abnormally high ceruloplasmin and oxidase levels [4]. However, these researchers considered dietary factors, liver damage and chronic infections as possible contributory factors. Meanwhile, preliminary experiments were indicating that excitement tends to elevate ceruloplasmin. Normal people receiving a synthetic hallucinatory drug demonstrated the same elevated ceruloplasmin as psychotic schizophrenics. Other workers were unable to find significant differences in ceruloplasmin oxidase activity in schizophrenic children and adults as compared with controls [5,6,7].

In 1962, Dr. Michael Briggs of Wellington, New Zealand theorised that many cases of 'schizophrenia' were really cases of chronic copper poisoning. The theory was based on the higher copper levels found in many schizophrenics which explained altered body chemistry [8].

In the next decade, research into copper accelerated and more and more evidence accumulated to confirm the copper connection. But not all studies were positive. What was the missing factor? Out of twenty groups of scientists who have studied copper levels in schizophrenics, fifteen considered 'schizophrenia' as a homogeneous clinical entity. Only four groups of scientists allowed for the possibility that 'simplistic schizophrenia' as a homogeneous clinical entity. Only four groups of scientists allowed for the possibility that 'simplistic schizophrenia' is a diagnosis made out of reluctant desperation. We had found that a sub-group of about 50 percent of our diagnosed 'schizophrenic' patients were high in copper. These patients often experienced paranoia and hallucinations. With nutritional therapy designed to reduce the copper burden of the body, the paranoia and hallucinations improved. The antidote was extra zinc, or zinc and manganese. Unlike many researchers, we did not study the hodgepodge 'simplistic schizophrenia' but studied each patient in depth over many months and years with a blood tests taken for copper, zinc, manganese and many other biochemical markers at each visit. Some of our patients have been studied for twenty years.

Niacin Lowers Copper

The histapenic patient has many similarities to pellagra patients. Pellagra, caused by B3 deficiency, was prevalent in the Southern States of America in the 1940s. Doctors Finddlay and Venter found that pellagra sufferers were also high in copper [9]. In India in 1974, Doctor Krishnammachavi studied copper in pellagra patients and found an abnormally high level which dropped with niacin (B3) treatment [10]. These findings, backed up by the fact that hair copper and urinary excretion of copper are also high in this vitamin deficient state, indicated that B3 deficiency causes copper levels to rise, making B3 another potential antidote to copper.

Vitamin C Deficiency Raises Copper Levels

Dr. Yvonne Hitier of France studied copper levels in guinea pigs on a diet deficient in vitamin C [11]. As the animals become C-deficient, the copper levels in the blood serum rose steadily until a level 2.5 times higher than normal was reached at death. This is a vicious circle in that high copper levels are known to destroy vitamin C. This may, in part, explain why the early treatment of mental illness with large doses of vitamins B3 and C often helped patients.

Two tentative conclusions might be drawn: High copper may produce a mental illness similar to that of B3-deficiency pellagra.The combined deficiency of both vitamins B3 and C may synergistically raise copper levels.

The Birth Control Pill Raises Copper

It is a well established fact that ceruloplasmin, the copper-containing protein, is produced faster in the presence of the female hormone, oestrogen, and women taking contraceptive pills uniformly exhibit raised copper levels. It is also interesting to note that any biological state which elevates the serum copper is apt to increase the need of vitamin C. So both mental illness, late pregnancy and particularly the use of the contraceptive pill produce states of elevated copper levels, which in turn may aggravate depression and disperception in schizophrenic patients on the pill. Animals given oestrogen show a marked reduction in blood levels of vitamin C. For women, vitamin C levels are highest at ovulation and lowest during menstruation, so cyclical problems may again be tied in with copper and vitamin C.

In summary, high levels of copper can cause mental illness, often characterised by extreme fears, paranoia and hallucinations. The copper may be the result of drinking water passing through copper pipes, copper pots and pans, the contraceptive pill and even copper IUDs. Or it can be the result of vitamin C or B3 deficiency. Either way, copper lowers histamine and as histamine levels return to normal so does the individual.

16

NIACIN THERAPY – A CURE FOR SCHIZOPHRENIA?

In October of 1990 a 24 year old woman arrived in my office. Six months earlier she began to hallucinate and become paranoid. During three weeks in hospital she was started on a tranquilliser. For several months after a premature discharge, she almost starved until a retired physician took her into her home to feed her. When I saw her she still suffered visual hallucinations, but no longer heard voices. I started her on 3 grams of niacin and 3 grams of vitamin C, daily. Three days later she was much better. By February 1991 she was well. By February 1995 she no longer needed drugs. She is still well and lives with her sister. (Case history supplied from Dr Abram Hoffer.)

One of the classic vitamin deficiency diseases is pellagra. Due to vitamin B3 (niacin) deficiency, the classic symptoms are the '3D's' - dermatitis diarrhoea and dementia. A more extensive list of symptoms might include headaches, sleep disturbance, hallucinations, thought disorder, anxiety and depression. The amino acid tryptophan can be converted into niacin. A lack of tryptophan, a lack of niacin, or both can trigger pellagra. At the turn of this century, there were said to be 25,000 cases annually in the US, focussed in the southern states where corn, lacking in tryptophan, was a staple food.

Officially it doesn't really exist any more in the civilised world due to improved nutrition and the fortification of foods with niacin. Yet, this year alone I have seen four possible cases of probable pellagra. The first two, both girls, had been diagnosed with schizophrenia. When asked what other symptoms they recalled at the time they started to feel mentally unwell, both remembered loose bowels and eczema or

113

Will niacin therapy help you?

Do you have the following characteristics?

1 A recent diagnosis of mental illness
2 Visual of auditory hallucinations or illusions
3 Anxiety or paranoia
4 Loose bowels or skin problems when the illness started
5 Mental confusion and inability to think straight
6 Depression
7 Personality deterioration

If the majority of the above apply you may benefit from:

- Niacin, 'no-flush' niacin or niacinamide 1,000mg (1 gram) twice a day
- Vitamin C, 1 gram after each meal
- plus a basic supplement programme (see page 198)

dermatitis. At the time, their doctors and psychiatrists didn't make the connection. I doubt many doctors or specialists even hold the possibility of nutrient deficiency on their check list of causes of so-called schizophrenia. One was proven B3 deficient by tests and responded well. The other, five years on from the initial onset, no longer tested deficient and responded less well to supplementation.

Two other cases illustrate another important point. In this case, two male teenagers, both diagnosed as schizophrenia and hospitalised, didn't have the associated symptoms of diarrhoea and dermatitis. Both responded so well to 1,000 to 2,000mg of niacin (100 times the RDA) that, within days they both became lucid, were discharged and have continued to improve, requiring less or no medication. From their diets one wouldn't suspect they had been chronically deficient in vitamin B3, yet their body chemistry responded to 100 times the amount needed by most. Some practitioners call this 'vitamin dependency', but we are all vitamin dependent. It's just that some people need more, perhaps for genetic reasons, that others.

Niacin Therapy

The use of 'megadoses' of niacin was first tried by Drs Humphrey Osmond and Abram Hoffer in 1951. So impressed were they with the results of acute schizophrenics that, in 1953, they ran the first double-blind therapeutic trials in the history of psychiatry. Their first two trials showed significant improvement giving at least 3 grams (3,000mg) a day, compared to placebos [1,2].

They also found that chronic schizophrenics, not first-time sufferers but long-term in-patients, showed little improvement. The results of six double blind controlled trials showed that the natural recovery rate was doubled. Later they found that chronic patients treated up to seven years in combination with other nutrients showed a 60 per cent recovery rate.

Over the next twenty years over a dozen trials tested the effects of niacin therapy with variable results, however all tested the effects on chronic patients, except for one researcher, Dr Wittenberg. His first trial showed no significant difference [3]. In the second trial he too found improvement in the acute schizophrenics, confirming the effectiveness of niacin therapy. However, the psychiatric community paid little attention to Wittenberg's second study and declared niacin therapy ineffective on the basis on the non-response of previous short trials showing no effect with chronic patients, confirming Hoffer and Osmond's earlier research.

Since then Dr Hoffer has published ten year follow-ups on schizophrenics treated with niacin, compared to those not treated with niacin. In the niacin patients there were substantially fewer admissions, days in hospital and suicides. He continues to treat acute schizophrenics with niacin and reports a 90% cure rate in acute schizophrenics who follow his nutritional programme. The former Director of Psychiatric Research in Saskatchewan in Canada defines cure as symptom-free, able to socialise with friends and family, and paying income tax!

Having recorded 4,000 cases and published double-blind trials Dr Hoffer is convinced that this approach is a major breakthrough in the treatment of mental illness.

Niacin Theories

Just how niacin works is still unsolved. Knowing that people with schizophrenia had hallucinations, seeing and hearing things, Hoffer worked out that the stress hormone adrenalin can be turned into adrenochrome, a chemical known to induce hallucinations. Being a biochemist he deduced that giving large amounts of vitamin B3 would prevent the formation of adrenochrome. B3 has many other important functions in cells which could also explain its effects.

Niacin also helps to raise abnormally low histamine levels, and detoxifies copper, both of which are related to mental illness. Niacin is also needed to turn essential fatty acids into prostaglandins. These, in turn, are needed to help balance neurotransmitter levels in the brain. The neurotransmitter serotonin is also made from tryptophan in the presence of enough niacin. So there are many possible ways this vitamin could affect brain function.

Hoffer also found that patients who tested positive for pyroluria (see next chapter) were more likely to respond while, at the Princeton Bio Center, Pfeiffer found that 'high histamine' patients didn't respond the high doses of niacin, and sometimes got worse. So large doses of niacin are most likely to be effective for acute not chronic schizophrenics who are not histadelic, are pyroluric and have some of the classic low histamine symptoms of hallucinations, anxiety and thought disorder. However, even histadelics can benefit from a lower intake of niacin at around 50mg a day.

Is it Safe?

The amount of niacin that's needed is around 2 to 4 grams a day. A minimum therapeutic level is 1 gram a day. These levels are in the order of one hundred times the RDA. Levels of niacin much higher than these, particularly in sustained release tablets, can be toxic, causing liver damage [4]. Out of perhaps 100,000 people taking megadoses of niacin over the past forty years there have been two deaths due to liver failure. In a third jaundice occurred from a slow release preparation. When the same patient was placed back on standard niacin he no longer got jaundice. In any event, even these levels are best taken under the supervision of a qualified practitioner.

Niacin comes in different forms. Niacin (formerly known as nicotinic

116

acid) causes a blushing sensation, accompanied with increase in skin temperature and slight itching. This effect lasts for up to 30 minutes. However, if 500mg or 1,000mg of niacin are taken twice a day at regular intervals the blushing stops.

Some supplement companies produce a 'no-flush' niacin by binding niacin with inositol. This works and avoids the blush, which is not harmful. It is probably the best form but is more expensive. Niacin also comes in the form of niacinamide which doesn't cause blushing and is good for people who don't like the blushing effect. Niacin, however, has the advantage of lowering cholesterol.

17

PYROLURIA - THE ZINC LINK

Since she was 11, Sara's life had been a nightmare of mental and physical suffering. Her history included chronic insomnia, episodic loss of reality, attempted suicide by hanging, amnesia, partial seizures, nausea, vomiting and loss of periods. Her knees were so painful (X-rays showed poor cartilages) and her mind so disperceptive that she walked slowly with her feed wide apart like a peasant following a hand plough drawn by tired oxen. Psychiatrists at three different hospitals gave the dubious waste-basket labels of 'schizophrenia', 'paranoid schizophrenia' and 'schizophrenia with convulsive disorder'. At times her left side went into spasms with foot clawed and fist doubled up. Both arm and leg had a wild flaying motion. Restraints were needed at these times. Psychotherapy was ineffective and most tranquillisers accentuated the muscle symptoms. She tested positive for pyroluria and was given B6 and zinc.

Urinary kryptopyrrole was at times as high as 1000mcg%, the normal range being less than 15. She was diagnosed as B6 and zinc deficient and treatment was started. Over three months her knees became normal, the depression subsided, as did the seizures, her periods returned, the nausea vanished and so did the abdominal pain. She has had no recurrence of her grave illness, finished college and now works in New York. She takes zinc and B6 daily. When under stress of any kind, she increases her intake of vitamin B6.

Perhaps the most significant discovery in the nutritional treatment of mental illness is that many depressed and mentally ill people are deficient in vitamin B6 and zinc. But this deficiency is no ordinary deficiency that is simply corrected by eating more foods that are rich in zinc and B6. It is connected with the abnormal production of

Are you pyroluric?

Do you have disperceptions and some of the following?
 1 Intolerance to some protein foods, alcohol or drugs
 2 Definite breath and body odour
 3 Morning nausea and constipation
 4 Difficulty remembering your dreams
 5 Crowded upper front teeth
 6 White spots on your finger nails
 7 Pale skin which doesn't tolerate sunlight
 8 Frequent upper abdominal pain
 9 Frequent head colds and infections
10 Stretch marks in the skin
11 Irregular menstrual cycle or impotency
12 Any of the above when stressed
13 You belong to an all-girl family with look-alike sisters

If a majority of the above apply you may benefit from:
• Vitamin B6 100mg, am and pm - enough for nightly dream recall (do not exceed 1,000mg!)
• Zinc 30mg, am and pm.
• Manganese 10mg, am and pm.
• plus a basic supplement programme (see page 198)

a group of chemicals called 'pyrroles'. A patient with a high level of pyrroles in the urine needs more B6 and zinc, since these pyrroles rob the body of these essential nutrients. About 30% of schizophrenics have 'pyroluria', and 11% of 'normals' have it as well.

Closely ranked in creativity to the compulsive productivity of the histadelic patient is the 'pyroluric' patient. Many great people in history have shown the signs of pyroluria. Among these are the poet, Emily Dickinson and the scientific philosopher and discoverer, Charles Darwin. Their life stories reflect many of the character traits associated with this condition.

Pyroluria Linked with Withdrawal and Seclusion

Reflections on the meaning of life and death were the two major influences in the life works of both Emily Dickinson and Charles Darwin. Their literary and scientific contributions have been praised for over a century, but only recently has science begun to look into their secluded lives and gather the pertinent data that suggests that Emily Dickinson and Charles Darwin may have suffered biochemical abnormalities which produced the physical and psychiatric symptoms of pyroluria.

They both possessed great originality and drive. Because of this creativity they feared and avoided any outside stress that might upset their delicate balance of emotion and ideas. Any change in routine or involvement with people outside the family group provoked stress which could manifest itself as a tremor, palpitations, insomnia and (for Darwin) nausea and vomiting as well. As Darwin and Dickinson approached the age of 30 they purposely chose voluntary exile. Emily was succinctly subjective when she wrote, 'The soul selects her own society then shuts the door'.

An amalgam of pyroluric symptoms manifested themselves during the course of their isolated lives. They shared bouts of depression, blinding headaches, nervous exhaustion, a change of handwriting and a familial dependence. Darwin endured, usually without complaint, a crippling fatigue and loss of appetite and underwent such extreme depression that it pained him to look at a printed page. Emily became hypersensitive to normal daylight and suffered such extreme eye pains that she, too, could not read.

Medical and psychological authorities have claimed emotional, psychological or simple physical reasons for the reclusiveness of Dickinson and Darwin. For them, seclusion may have been a means by which they could combat the distressing symptoms of pyroluria. A cloistered life provided them with regulated daily routine and diet, adequate rest and, most important, the avoidance of stressful situations and experiences that enabled them to continue their brilliant studies and productive writing. Emily Dickinson gave her personal explanation when she wrote 'Insanity for the sane seems so unreasonable'.

Because of her strict seclusion, medical data on Emily Dickinson is scant. We do know that Emily only wore white dresses. Both Dickinson and Darwin worshipped their protective fathers, and were severely grieved by their fathers' deaths. As they slipped deeper into seclusion, their handwriting changed and became less legible. When young, both Dickinson and Darwin enjoyed the company of friends and going to parties. However, as they grew older they became retiring and avoided even the closest friends, except through correspondence. Certainly pyroluria occurs in our most original psychiatric patients and therefore deserves first consideration as an explanation when the illnesses of Emily Dickinson and Charles Darwin are reviewed.

How Pyroluria was Discovered

The first time urinary excretion of pyrroles was connected with psychosis was in 1958, when a Canadian doctor, Dr. Payza, noted a new substance in the urine of several patients undergoing experimental LSD model psychosis. The abnormal chemical found in the urine of these patients was later found in the urine of many psychiatric patients who had never taken LSD or any other drug. In 1961, Drs. Abram Hoffer and Mahon found the 'mauve factor' in 27 out of 39 schizophrenic patients. (The extracted urine made a lavender colour when reacted with Ehrlich's Reagent.) One-third of the psychiatric patients with diagnosis other than 'schizophrenia' also had the mauve factor in their urine. In 1963, Drs Hoffer and Osmond coined the word 'malvaria' to designate mauve positive patients. O'Reilly and Hughes (1965), studying normal and psychiatric patients, found the mauve factor in 11% normal, 24% of disturbed children, 42% of psychiatric patients and 52% of schizophrenics. But the scientist who really solved the mauve factor enigma was Donald Irvine of Saskatoon in Canada[1]. He found the exact structure of the mauve factor to be the chemical, kryptopyrrole, which was then confirmed by Dr Arthur Sohler of the Princeton Bio Center[2]. We suggested that kryptopyrrole would produce a severe B6 deficiency (since pyrroles bind to aldehydes, and pyridoxal (B6) is an aldehyde). This was confirmed and we further found that the complex of pyridoxal with kryptopyrrole took excess zinc out of the body.

With this knowledge, effective therapy was at hand and the mauve factor patients got well when treated with both vitamin B6 and zinc.

With this discovery the term 'pyroluria' was coined. Since 1971 we have seen thousands of pyroluric patients, both at the Princeton Bio Center and at the Institute for Optimum Nutrition in London, and most of them have responded well to B6 and zinc therapy. Other nutrients are also important as nutrients work in synergy. For example, vitamin B3 and B6 are synergistic, and Dr Hoffer has reported excellent results with niacin (B3) therapy.

The Signs and Symptoms of Pyroluria

The signs and symptoms of pyroluria are many. There seems to be a genetic or familial component. A family history of mental illness or suicide, all-girl families with male children miscarried are all possible signs. Consider the story of one of our patients.

A pyroluric doctor married a pyroluric nurse. The outcome of the marriage was four children and three miscarriages. One of the miscarriages was a boy. The sex of the other two was never determined. Four daughters lived, but by the age of 20, three of them had been labelled schizophrenic. With these labels we have the possibility of three walking corpses out of a family, the boys are miscarried or stillborn, or have birth defects, while the daughters live normally until stressed at the age of 15-20 years. With stress, the daughters will have psychiatric difficulties and this usually occurs in the last years of school or the first years of college. The stress may cause depression (suicide) or disperceptions and hallucinations.

Pyroluria is a stress-related condition and when symptoms are brought on by stress pyroluria should be considered. Most adults can predict and recognise stress in their lives. For the child the parent must recognise stressful situations and, if possible, circumvent the stress. The stressful time for teenagers may be the first love affair, either homo or heterosexual (loss of virginity, homosexual panic), or the act of of leaving home to live in a dormitory in college. Joining the armed forces is stressful and may precipitate illness if the patient is pyroluric.

Pyrolurics often have weak immune systems and may suffer from frequent ear infections as a child as well as colds, fevers and chills. Neurological symptoms include fatigue, nervous exhaustion, insomnia, poor memory, hyperactivity, seizures, poor learning ability, confusion, an inability to think clearly, depression and mood swings.

There can be impotence in males or lack of regular periods in females. The pyroluric often has bad breath and a strange body odour, cannot tolerate alcohol or drugs, may wake up with nausea, have cold hands and feet and abdominal pain. Not all these symptoms are present in all pyrolurics, however a number of these symptoms should make you suspicious.

The Zinc and B6 Connection

During 1967 and 1971, when we were vigorously applying vitamins to patients, we found that some young patients improved rapidly although they were neither high nor low in blood histamine. We were also measuring pyrroles in their urine and finally came to the conclusion that these young patients improved as the pyrrole levels decreased and the dose of vitamin B6 was increased. The patients were on zinc supplements since we knew that histamine was stored with zinc in the terminal buds of the nerve cells. Later in 1971 the dramatic case of Sara, described at the start of this chapter, provided the necessary data to link pyroluria with zinc and B6 deficiency. We learned many facts about pyroluria as we got Sara well over a period of three months:

1   Her knees needed adequate zinc and manganese to develop normal cartilage and tendons.

2   Her brain needed adequate B6 to prevent the abnormal messages which cause convulsive seizures.

3   Her brain was alive with abnormal cross-talk between neurons which gave the final behaviour of depression, amnesia and disperceptions.

4   Her bone marrow produced inadequate synthesis of haemoglobin resulting in anaemia on pyrroles in her urine.

5   Her endocrine glands required adequate zinc and B6 to establish a normal menstrual cycle.

6   Her spleen and liver (like other patients with rupture of red cells) became engorged periodically with red cell debris to produce a severe upper abdominal pain. Sara walked completely bent over when she had this pain.

7   Sara (like the B6 pregnant woman) had nausea each morning when she did not get her morning dose of vitamin B6.

8   Sara (like a class of patients labelled schizophrenic) had a fruity odour to her breath and sweat.

9   Sara reacted adversely to tranquillisers and barbiturates because her tissue enzymes were B6 deficient and could not detoxify the drugs.

Mark Vonnegut (the son of Kurt Vonnegut) wrote Eden Express after recovery from pyroluria. Mark was stricken with insomnia which led to 'crazes' while in college. His book must be read to learn the difficulties that the patient encounters in mental hospitals. Mark had severe pyroluria when tested at the Princeton Bio Center in February 1973. He showed the usual rapid improvement when given daily zinc and enough B6 to produce dream recall. The big event of 1973 was our discovery that B6-deficient patients had no dream recall. with adequate B6 they remember the last dream of the night. With too much B6, a patient may awaken every two hours during the whole night with vivid dreams - and remember up to four dreams in the morning.

Dream recall is Normal

Knowing that we are concerned with nutrition and chemistry, some patients have a perplexed look when we ask about dream recall. Some say they have not dreamed enough to be able to tell their dreams at the breakfast table. Not so! Many original adults will use their dreams to revitalise their minds and their daily productivity. For instance, Dave Brubeck, the musician, told us that in his younger days he got ideas for musical composition from dreams. For a period the dreams vanished but now with adequate daily B6 intake, he has vivid dreams which again help his musical composition and complex arrangements.

When patients ask us why we want them to have better dream recall, I simply state, 'Dream recall is normal. We want you to be normal'. One pyroluric patient called excitedly to relate that the first new dream he had was about the terrible time he had had in the mental hospital (a real id catharsis). He asked if I had planned that for him. Because of my usually busy day I said 'Yes' and went on to the next dreamless patient.

Another 13-year old young lady who had only had nightmares in the last two years now found that she had pleasant dreams. Her only comment was that 'Some of my dreams are awfully sexy.' I responded by saying pragmatically that at least she wouldn't get pregnant from dreams. She replied, 'Oh! I wouldn't go that far even in my dreams!'

Yet another 17 year old patient had her nightmares changed to pleasant dreams. Her psychoanalyst protested that nightmares were useful for the elimination of inner aggression and that the change to pleasant dreams was a step backwards! I sided with the patient who liked the pleasant dreams. Others apply our findings to diagnose and help the pyroluric. At least twenty clinics around the USA and a few in Europe do pyrrole testing of the urine and carry out zinc and B6 treatment with pyroluric patients. A few orthodox clinics are having success, as reported in the medical journals.

'Zinc Deficiency Presenting as Schizophrenia' is the title of an article published by Drs. Stanton, Donald and Green, in Current Psychiatric Digest, in December 1976 3. These doctors work at the Psychiatric Institute of Columbia, South Carolina and point out the need to study zinc and copper relationships in psychotic patients.

Their zinc-deficient psychiatric patient was an 18 year old teenager from Carolina, off to college as a music major in California. Under social stress at college he became agitated and when admitted to a California medical centre was found to be disorientated as to time and place and bothered by constant visual and auditory hallucinations. He did not respond to medication (Prolixon and Haldol). He returned to South Carolina and was committed into a mental hospital for further study and treatment. The only laboratory abnormality among the routine tests was elevation of the liver enzymes SGOT, SGPT and LDH, all of which rise with B6 deficiency. Other drugs were tried without success. He had episodes of elevated blood pressure, 150/120 - a sign of copper excess. He was delusional, hallucinating, self-destructive and when questioned he slowly repeated the words of the examining doctor. A series of fifteen electroconvulsive shock treatments (ECT) were given with some temporary improvements but within ten days of the ECT the patient was back to the original psychotic baseline and attempted to jump through a window.

When all else failed, trace metal levels were run on his blood serum. The zinc was 65mcg% (our normal being 100-120) and copper was 185 (our normal being 100mcg% for males). In the words of the authors: 'Because all other treatment had proven ineffective it was decided to treat the patient as if he were pyroluric and attempt to replace the zinc and B6.'

On 160mg zinc sulphate per day and 1000mg B6 twice a day, the patient became quiet in 2 days. He was more alert and was able to leave his locked room and join other patients in the ward. His muscle rigidity and tremor lessened. Progress was steady and within one month the patient was emotionally normal, making plans for the future and fully cogniscient of the world about him. His tested degree of insanity (In-patient behaviour scale) went from a high of 71 to a normal of 10 at discharge. Follow-up at one year found him back at college and doing well, his zinc level was still low (75mcg%) but his copper level was normal at 90mcg%. The patient cooperates fully and continues to take his daily dose of zinc and B6.

The doctors conclude: 'We do believe that there exists a group of patients who have a zinc deficiency which, complicated by emotional stress, may present a schizophrenic picture. Because of the success and safety of the treatment, it would seem worthwhile to attempt to identify and treat such patients.' I can only say a fervent 'Amen! Let's do it'.

Pyrolics do Better on Vegetarian Diets

Vegetarians are usually thin and healthy, and fully one-third of the world's population are vegetarians because of religion and the high price of animal protein.

One patient from a southern city in the USA found that she could not eat any protein foods such as fish, chicken or red meat without developing unreality, dizziness and even hallucinations when she closed her eyes. Without fail, she was unduly suspicious of her companions when she ate meat - she had paranoia! She thought she had an allergy to all proteins and she therefore came to us for food-allergy testing but on the initial tests we found her to be pyroluric with a high pyrrole level in her urine. We next found her to be both zinc and B6 deficient, as are all pyroluric patients. Both zinc and B6 are needed by the body to handle protein foods. With adequate vitamin B6 plus zinc and manganese she found that she could tolerate proteins for the first time in years. Furthermore, she started losing her fat and excess body fluids as a result of the new nutrients. She lost 15 pounds in weight in the short period of 2 months. Her dresses began to fit again.

The point to this case is that many disperceptive teenagers, when stressed, find that abnormal mental symptoms increase after a protein meal. They do feel better on an all vegetarian diet .

Clues from Skin, Hair, Teeth and Nails

The pyroluric patient is often pale due to lack of skin pigment. This we have labelled a 'China Doll Appearance'. Zinc and B6 are needed to produce pigment in both skin and hair. A pyroluric black patient will have the lightest skin of all the family. People who have never been able to have a skin tan (except albinos) will tan normally on zinc and B6. Local depigmentation (vitiligo) does not, unfortunately, respond to zinc therapy. The lack of hair on the head, eyelashes and eye brows can frequently be corrected with B6 and zinc. The new hair will grow in the individual's natural colour, the same as before the deficiency occurred. We have seen prematurely grey hair return to black with zinc therapy. The loss of hair in the last month of pregnancy, and with the use of the pill, is due to high copper and low zinc levels produced by oestrogens.

The teeth in the upper jaw may be crowded unless the patient has had orthodontic treatment. This overcrowding shows when the patient smiles. The upper dental arch is narrow with overlapping incisors. The enamel of the teeth will be poor if the patient has been zinc deficient during the period of tooth formation. Drs. Curson and Losee find both copper and cadmium to be high in the enamel of decayed teeth compared with that in healthy teeth. Extra zinc is the antidote to high copper and cadmium levels in all tissues of the body. The gums may be red and retracted (pyorrhoea) where there is zinc deficiency. Good dental hygiene combined with zinc and B6 will make the gums grow normally again.

The fingernails are white and spotted, opaquely white and tissue paper thin in the pyroluric patient. the very thinness of the nails plus anxiety leads to active fingernail biting. The actual nails are no more solid than 'hang nails' and everyone occasionally tears at hang nails with the teeth. Small wonder nail biting occurs. As you know from that occasional blue spot under the nail, it takes 6 months to grow a new nail so the nails will be strong in six months with adequate intake of zinc and B6. We confidently predict the cessation of nail biting in six months and our prediction seldom fails. Small white spots may resolve with zinc but larger white spots require five to six months to grow out with the nail.

Acne, eczema and herpes (cold sores) may all respond to zinc and B6 therapy. The avoidance of chocolates, nuts and thiamine and supplementation with l-lysine also help get rid of herpes. Psoriasis is characterised by a high serum copper level so this may also respond to continued zinc and B6 therapy. The effective treatment of severe skin disease may require as much as 60mg of zinc given two to three times per day, but this sort of dose should only be taken under supervision.

Summary

The careful study of people of all ages will find that about 10% of a normal population have pyroluria which can cause symptoms when the patient is stressed. Among hospitalised schizophrenics the incidence of pyroluria will approach 30% or more.

Effective treatment is found in supplementing extra zinc and B6. The adult dose of elemental zinc is 30mg (equivalent to 300mg zinc gluconate) taken am and pm and enough vitamin B6 should be given to produce normal dream recall. It is best not to take more than 500mg without proper supervision. The avoidance of stress is also helpful.

Pyroluria can occur at any age, is familial, and can be the cause of mental retardation, minimal brain damage, epilepsy, hyperactivity, delinquency, amnesia and one type of so-called 'schizophrenia'.

18

HYPOGLYCEMIA - OVERSTRESSED OR UNDERNOURISHED?

David was diagnosed as suffering from schizophrenia at the age of 20, having suffered from acute depression, paranoia and extreme mental confusion. He was also seeing and hearing things. He was put on the drug Stelazine which calmed him down, but he felt disoriented and couldn't go back to college or relate with friends and family in a normal way. He went to see a nutrition counsellor who identified that he was chronically deficient in vitamin B6 and zinc and had hypoglycemia. Within days of adding B6 and zinc supplements, changing his diet and avoiding sugar, coffee and alcohol he became symptom free. He was able to stop taking Stelazine and is now doing very well at University without any recurrence of his previous mental health problems.

The desire to eat sweet foods is prevalent in most societies all over the world. Sugar comes in many forms, from its most natural and wholesome packaging in fresh fruit to pure white table sugar, one of its most refined manifestations. Alcohol usually also contains a high sugar content. Stimulants are likewise universally popular. Nicotine in cigarettes and caffeine from tea, coffee, cocoa, cola drinks and chocolate are part of many people's daily routine. Most people would consider consumption of one or more of these as a normal part of everyday life. So why should there be a cause for concern? Everybody does it. It must be OK. Not so. Evidence is accumulating that excess sugar and stimulants has a disturbing effect on mental and emotional health by disrupting the balance of blood sugar, the brain's fuel.

There is a very important balancing act operating in the body by which a stable glucose or blood sugar level is maintained in the bloodstream. This is crucial in providing us with an even supply of energy for both body and mind. The brain relies completely on a continuous supply of glucose from the blood in order to work properly, with 30 per cent of available glucose being used as brain fuel. When glucose drops too low the brain immediately suffers, resulting in symptoms ranging from weakness, fatigue, faintness, dizziness, nervousness, irritability and trembling to anxiety, depression, forgetfulness, disruptive outbursts, confusion, difficulty concentrating, palpitations and blackouts. The term used to describe this difficulty with glucose control is glucose intolerance or hypoglycemia. It is estimated that as many as 1 in 4 people suffer from symptoms of glucose intolerance. Studies in prisons have found almost all offenders to have glucose intolerance [1]. A high intake of stimulants such as tea, coffee, sugar and cigarettes is frequently reported in mental institutions, where hypoglyecmia is the rule, rather than the exception.

It is the carbohydrate component in our diet which is digested and absorbed into the bloodstream as glucose. The pancreas responds to the arrival of the glucose into the blood by producing insulin which aids the transport of glucose into body cells for energy production, thereby stabilising blood glucose levels. When blood glucose drops considerably, for example after a long time without food, the adrenal glands are stimulated to release adrenaline and other hormones which act to normalise blood glucose levels by releasing glucose from the liver. Unfortunately, this elegant mechanism can easily be disturbed by the excessive use of sugar and stimulants, which trigger adrenaline release, with symptoms of glucose intolerance as a likely outcome. When sugary foods, alcohol or other highly refined carbohydrates are consumed frequently, the pancreas begins to over-react by producing too much insulin so that glucose drops below its optimum level. The adrenals become exhausted in their continuous attempts to boost blood glucose. Symptoms of glucose intolerance set in and a vicious cycle is created as more sugar is craved to relieve the symptoms. Caffeine and nicotine work in a similar way. They encourage glucose intolerance by their stimulant effect on the adrenals, creating a glucose high, followed by a sharp drop and inevitable craving. In time the adrenals become depleted, glucose intolerance becomes entrenched and physical, mental and emotional energy suffers.

Are you glucose intolerant?

Do you have disperceptions and
1 Weakness, fatigue, faintness and dizziness
2 Nervousness, irritability, trembling and anxiety
3 Depression, forgetfulness, confusion and difficulty
   concentrating
4 Palpitations or blackouts

If a majority of the above apply you may benefit from:
• Avoidance of the junk foods, sugar, alcohol and white bread
• Regular exercise
• Manganese 10mg am and pm
• Zinc 15mg am and pm
• Chromium 200mcg a day
• plus a basic supplement programme (see page 198)

Symptoms of glucose intolerance can range from the mildly uncomfortable to the severely debilitating. Dr Carl Pfeiffer has classified glucose intolerance as one of the five main underlying factors in schizophrenia. Psychiatric symptoms of glucose intolerance have been noted to include unsocial or anti–social behaviour, phobias, suicide attempts, nervous breakdown and psychosis. In addition, studies have implicated sugar as a factor in the following conditions connected with mental and emotional health: aggressive behaviour [2,3,4,5,6,7], anxiety, attention–deficit [8] and hyperactivity, depression [9], eating disorders [10], fatigue [11], learning disabilities [12,13,14,15] and PMS. Caffeine has been implicated in fatigue [16], anxiety [17,18], depression [19], PMS, insomnia [20,21] psychotic episode and increased psychotic symptoms in schizophrenics [22].

A High Complex Carbohydrate Diet Works Best

Nutritionists and nutritionally-oriented doctors have traditionally prescribed a high protein, low carbohydrate diet for their hypoglycemic patients, with an emphasis on frequent meals and snacks. Such a diet often included large quantities of animal protein, and excluded carbohydrate-containing foods such as whole grains and fruits. Today we know that a diet low in saturated fat but rich in the essential fats, low in protein, high in complex carbohydrates and with plenty of water, gives consistently better results.

The key is the emphasis on complex carbohydrates - not the pure white sugar so many people find addictive, but the type of carbohydrates found in vegetables, nuts, seeds and whole grains (such as oatmeal). When used as the core of the hypoglycemic diet, these naturally occurring carbohydrates help regulate blood sugar levels, thus preventing the rapid swings responsible for hypoglycemic symptoms. These whole foods also contain the trace minerals necessary for the transport and utilisation of carbohydrates once inside the body.

While complex carbohydrate foods, such as wholegrains or beans, release their sugar content slowly, not all simple carbohydrates are fast releasing. Most fruit contains a different kind of sugar, fructose, which is also slow releasing. Increasing 'slow releasing' sugar foods, and reducing or avoiding 'fast releasing' sugar foods (see chart on page 47) and stimulants rapidly corrects glucose intolerance. Frequent meals and regular exercise also help to regulate glucose control.

Sugar Cannot be Used Without Minerals

Many vitamins and trace elements, including vitamin C, the B complex of vitamins, calcium, potassium, magnesium, zinc, chromium, manganese and phosphorus, are involved in glucose metabolism and the activities of the endocrine glands. The recently discovered Glucose Tolerance Factor (GTF) which contains chromium, is essential for proper carbohydrate metabolism. So too are B complex vitamins and C.

Testing for Glucose Intolerance

Gross blood sugar problems can be diagnosed from a blood or urine glucose test after an ingestion of sugar, such as a can of a sugared fizzy drink. More sensitive is a blood test measuring glycosylated haemoglobin. This is the extent by which the red blood cells have become 'sugar-coated' from a general excess of glucose in the blood. An alternative test is the five-hour glucose tolerance test. This method involves fasting for twelve hours, then ingesting glucose. At hourly or half-hourly intervals a blood sample is taken and tested for glucose . This shows how the individual responds to an ingestion of sugar.

For mineral levels hair analysis is probably the most versatile of the diagnostic tests. If you eat junk food, the body runs low on zinc, manganese and chromium, and other minerals mobilised to use and store the excess glucose. The hair analysis of such a hypoglycemic patient will therefore show low zinc, manganese and chromium.

Other Causes for Hypoglycemia

Impaired glucose metabolism engendered by disease is classified as organic or fasting hypoglycemia, since symptoms become more pronounced when food is withheld. An insulin secreting tumour of the pancreatic islet cells produces severe fasting hypoglycemia. Congenital liver enzyme defects, liver damage produced by alcohol, tobacco or infection, encephalitis, brain tumours, hypopituitarism and Addison's disease (an exhaustion of the adrenals) also cause it. These diseases are rare, accounting for only a few of the hypoglycemic disorders.

Defects in glucose metabolism resulting from secondary factors occur with far greater frequency. Such disorders are classified as nutritional, functional, reactive or fed hypoglycemia, because symptoms develop in response to food intake. Alimentary hypoglycemia, one type of nutritional glycemia, often develops in patients who undergo subtotal gastrectomy for peptic ulcers, as foods pass more rapidly into the small intestine when part of the stomach has been removed. Most often, prolonged stress, particularly the internal disturbance provoked by poor eating habits, triggers hypoglycemia.

Stress & Blood Sugar

Any physical or emotional trauma, such as pain, overexertion, childbearing, anxiety, grief, or fear causes the adrenal gland to release adrenalin, prompting an increase in blood glucose to supply the extra energy needed to deal with the stress. When a person suffers continual stress, the adrenal gland must constantly supply adrenalin. Eventually, this persistent demand exhausts the adrenal gland. When challenged, it can no longer produce enough adrenalin and hypoglycemia results.

Empty calories stress the pancreas and adrenal glands. When repeatedly forced to handle large amounts of glucose (derived from a diet rich in refined sugars), the pancreas becomes oversensitised and hypoglycemia develops. Every time glucose enters the blood, the pancreas over-reacts, releasing too much insulin which causes the cells to absorb and utilise glucose at top speed. The adrenal glands, striving to maintain proper glucose balance, become exhausted. Soon after a meal, blood sugar falls below fasting levels and the body craves sugar, producing the symptoms of hypoglycemia. Another dose of sugar relieves the symptoms for a short time, so many hypoglycemics nibble continually on sweets, without minerals, a pattern which only aggravates the underlying metabolic disorder.

Low Blood Pressure and Low Body Temperature

A distinctive characteristic of hypoglycemia is low blood pressure and lowered body temperature. Hypoglycemia often complain of cold hands and feet and many experience cold sweats. Dr Freinkel (1972) and Dr Molar (1974) studied hypothermia in laboratory-induced hypoglycemia and found significant decreases in body temperature associated with the onset of other hypoglycemic symptoms. Both doctors attribute this phenomenon to the effect of glucose deficiency on brain cells, since the hypothalamus controls body temperature. Many doctors note the low blood pressure but shrug it off with 'Well, you'll never die of high blood pressure'. A normal blood pressure is needed to keep the hands warm and the mind alert. Manganese raises blood pressure and all hypoglycemic patients are deficient in manganese.

Hypoglycemia is Easy to Treat

For many 'diseases of lifestyle' the outlook is grim but not so for hypoglycemia. All that is needed for the disease to go away is a change in lifestyle. A change to a 'caveman's diet', high in complex carbohydrate, together with daily exercise will not only do away with some symptoms but also make all the tests go negative - to such an extent that the hospital doctor may say, 'See your glucose tolerance test is normal, you never had that mythical disease called hypoglycemia!' You should know better since you have cured yourself by eating the foods with natural minerals, by taking proper mineral and vitamin supplements, and by exercising to your tolerance each day.

19

THE ALLERGY CONNECTION

Janet was diagnosed with manic depression at the age of 15. At times she would become hyperactive and manic, and at other times become completely depressed. She was put on three drugs - Lithium, Tegretol and Zirtek. These helped control the severity of her manic phases, but she was still frequently depressed and anxious. Two years later she consulted a nutrition counsellor who found she was deficient in many nutrients, especially zinc, and allergic to wheat. As soon as her nutrient deficiencies were corrected and she stopped eating wheat her health rapidly improved. She was able to stop all medication and, provided she stays off wheat, no longer gets depressed. She is now doing her final degree exams and continues to feel good and achieve well. However, if she has any wheat, even inadvertently in a sauce, she becomes depressed, confused, forgetful and anxious for 3 to 4 days. Her manic phases, however, have never returned.

The idea that food affects the mind is an alien concept to many people. But since the brain is perhaps the most delicate organ of the body, using sometimes as much as 30% of all the energy we derive from food, this should be no surprise. Allergies to food can upset levels of hormones and other key chemicals in the brain, resulting in symptoms ranging from depression to schizophrenia.

The knowledge that allergy to foods and chemicals can adversely affect moods and behaviour in susceptible individuals has been known for a very long time. Early reports, as well as current research, have found that allergies can affect any system of the body, including the central nervous system. They can cause a diversity of symptoms including fatigue, slowed thought processes, irritability, agitation, aggressive behaviour, nervousness, anxiety, depression, schizophrenia, hyperactivity and varied learning disabilities [1-8].Food intolerance, lack of absorption of food and relief with fasting are three key pointers to the food-allergic patient. These patients usually have a low blood histamine, a fast pulse and food idiosyncrasies which may be expressed as strong likes and dislikes. Favourite foods are often the offending foods so the patients is like an addict, eating the offending food to obtain a psychiatric high.

The allergic child may suffer from the so-called 'allergic-tension-fatigue syndrome' described by Dr. Frederic Speer in 1954 [9], which results in irritability, hyperactivity and impaired concentration, thus adversely affecting school performance. The most convincing evidence that this is indeed so, comes from a well conducted double–blind, placebo controlled crossover trial by Dr Egger and his team, who studied 76 hyperactive children to find out whether diet can contribute to behavioural disorders. The results showed that 79% of the children tested reacted adversely to artificial food colourants and preservatives, primarily to tartrazine and benzoic acid, which produced a marked deterioration in their behaviour.However no child reacted to these alone. In fact 48 different foods were found to produce symptoms among the children tested. For example 64% reacted to cow's milk, 59% to chocolate, 49% to wheat, 45% to oranges, 39% to eggs, 32% to peanuts, and 16% to sugar. Interestingly enough it was not only the children's behaviour which improved after the individual dietary modification. Most of the associated symptoms also improved considerably, such as headaches, fits, abdominal discomfort, chronic rhinitis, aches in limbs, skin rashes and mouth ulcers [10].

Another similar double–blind controlled food trial by Dr Egger and his team was conducted on 88 children suffering from frequent migraines. As before, most children reacted to several foods/chemicals. However the following foods/chemicals were found to be most prevalent: cows milk provoked symptoms in 27 children, egg in 24, chocolate in 22, both oranges and wheat in 21, benzoic acid in 14 and tartrazine in 12.

Yet again, interestingly enough, after dietary modification, not only migraines improved but also associated physical disorders such as abdominal pain, muscle aches, fits, rhinitis, recurrent mouth ulcers, asthma and eczema, as well as a variety of behavioural disorders [11].

While food dyes or additives may cause the symptoms, the most commonly implicated types of food are milk, wheat, egg, beef, corn, cane sugar and chocolate. A similar syndrome in adults has been called simply 'cerebral allergy'. The allergy often appears in a masked form, in which the individual actually feels better after ingesting a favourite food. However, in a variable number of hours a severe let-down occurs and the patient experiences symptoms which may be diffuse and non-specific and often include headache, depression, nasal stuffiness and sleepiness.

Allergies Run in Families

Allergy runs in families and so does cerebral allergy. The allergic diseases have many presenting symptoms and common names so that the infant who cannot tolerate cow's or goat's milk may be starting a life long fight against allergies called colic, eczema or croup. Lack of breast feeding may predispose the infant to allergies because the infant does not get the needed immune bodies from the mother. Colic may progress into coeliac disease wherein the food goes through the intestinal tract unchanged. If a sample of the intestinal wall is studied, it can be seen that the finger-like villi that absorb the food are missing and the intestinal wall is smooth and scarred. Asthma may occur and alternate with the other allergic diseases. Children eating food dyes or food naturally high in salicylates may develop hyperactivity.

Adults are also affected by food and/or chemical allergy.When Dr Philpott, a US allergy expert, examined 250 emotionally disturbed patients for a possible presence of food/chemical allergies, using an elimination and challenge diet, he found that the highest percentage of symptoms seemed to occur in patients diagnosed as psychotic 12. For example, out of 53 patients diagnosed as schizophrenic, 64% reacted adversely to wheat, 50% to cow's milk, 75% to tobacco and 30% to petrochemical hydrocarbons. The emotional symptoms caused by allergic intolerance ranged from mild central nervous system symptoms such as dizziness, blurred vision, anxiety, depression, tension, hyperactivity and speech difficulties to gross psychotic symptoms. At the same time, the individuals also experienced various adverse physical symptoms such as headaches, feelings of unsteadiness, weakness, palpitations and muscle aches and pains.

Do you have cerebral allergies?

Do you have disperceptions and
1 A history of infantile colic
2 A history of infantile eczema
3 A history of coeliac disease (malabsorption)
4 A history of asthma, rashes or hay fever
5 Favourite daily foods
6 Excessive daily mood swings
7 Frequent rapid colds
8 Seasonal allergies
9 Relief of symptoms with fasting
10 Intolerance to foods such as wheat or milk.

If a majority of the above apply you may benefit from:
• Methionine, 500mg, am and pm
• Calcium 500mg, am and pm
• Zinc 15mg, am and pm
• Manganese10mg , am and pm
• B6 adequate for dream recall (no more than 1,000mg)
• Vitamin C, 1000-2000mg, am and pm
• plus a basic supplement programme (see page 198)
  as well as testing for, and avoiding allergens

These studies are prime examples of how problems created by allergies often produce a multitude of physical and mental symptoms and affect many body symptoms. They not only can affect the central nervous system and the brain, but also usually affect the whole body in various ways. Furthermore these allergies are very specific for each individual, i.e. the same foods/chemicals hardly ever produce the same symptoms in different people. Therefore the diagnosis is often made by eliminating certain foods, then reintroducing them, one by one. If reactions occur, the diagnosis is positive. Elimination/challenge testing should always be done under expert supervision, particularly if symptoms include fits, asthma, schizophrenia or severe depression.

Here are a few examples of how this elimination and challenge diet have been used safely and effectively in treating people suffering from various mental health problems [13].

Experimental double-blind study:

Thirty patients suffering from anxiety, depression, confusion or difficulty in concentration were tested, using a placebo controlled trial, as to whether individual food allergies could really produce mental symptoms in these individuals. The results showed that allergies alone, not placebos, were able to produce the following symptoms: severe depression, nervousness, feeling of anger without a particular object, loss of motivation and severe mental blankness. The foods/chemicals which produced most severe mental reactions were wheat, milk, cane sugar, tobacco smoke and eggs [14].

Experimental control study:

Ninety-six patients diagnosed as suffering from alcohol dependence, major depressive disorders and schizophrenia were compared to 62 control subjects selected from adult hospital staff members for a possible food/chemical intolerance. The results showed that the group of patients diagnosed as depressives had the highest number of allergies, i.e. 80% were found to be allergic to barley and 100% were allergic to egg white. Over 50% of alcoholics tested were found to be allergic to egg white, milk, rye and barley. Out of the group of people diagnosed as schizophrenics 80% were found to be allergic to both milk and eggs. Only 9% of the control group were found to suffer from any allergies [15].

Experimental double–blind study:

Routinely treated schizophrenics, who on admission were randomly assigned to a diet free of cereal grain and milk while on the locked ward, were discharged from the hospital nearly twice as rapidly as control patients assigned to a high–cereal diet. Wheat gluten secretly added to the cereal–free diet abolished this effect, suggesting that wheat gluten may be a cause of schizophrenic symptoms in susceptible individuals [16].

Two recent reports estimate that 2 in every 10 people now suffer from allergies [17,18]. The young developing nervous system seems to be particularly vulnerable to any allergenic or toxic overload, leading frequently to various behavioural disorders such as hyperactivity and learning disabilities. A further survey estimates that at least 1 child in l0 may react adversely to some common foods and/or food additives[19].

It is an interesting fact that a great number of drugs used in today's psychiatry are very similar in composition to antihistamines, which are commonly used in the treatment of allergies. For example tricyclic and related antidepressant drugs, such as imipramine (Tofranil) and Amitriptyline are also known to suppress brain histamine receptors. In addition, the following drugs used in the treatment of psychosis and related disorders are also known to inhibit brain histamine production: phenothiazine derivatives, such as chlorpromazine (Largactil), promazine (Sparine), Thioridazine etc. Furthermore promethazine, which is used in the treatment of anxiety and related disorders, is also commonly used in the treatment of allergies [20]. The fact that antihistamine-like drugs are widely used in the treatment of various mental disorders suggests that some mental problems could indeed be allergenic in origin. This being the case, it would surely be prudent to suggest that, before any medication is prescribed, all individuals suffering from mental health conditions should always be screened for a possible food/chemical intolerance.

Nutritional Treatment is the Answer

Several vitamins are noted for their effectiveness in reducing allergic symptoms. Vitamins C and B6 are probably the most effective. Dr. William Philpott has used both of these vitamins intravenously to turn off allergic symptoms provoked by testing for allergies. The patients on adequate vitamin C will have fewer allergic symptoms. B6 should be given to the point of nightly dream recall and the minerals calcium and potassium should be in plentiful supply in the diet. Zinc and manganese are also needed by the allergic patient. Elimination of the offending foods may be needed for several months. For multiple food allergies, in which this approach would severely limit the diet, a four-day rotation diet in which each food is eaten only once every four days should be tried. If this approach is unsuccessful, intradermal allergy testing to determine the degree of allergy and the neutralising dose of each allergen is recommended.

Testing for Allergies

Intradermal testing, which is the method we use at the Princeton Bio Center, is based on reliable skin testing procedures that are controlled, sensitive and effective methods of diagnosing food and/or inhalant allergies. Diagnosing a specific allergy consists of an intradermal injection (under the top layer of skin of the upper arm) of the food or inhalant extract in varying dilutions to determine the exact degree of sensitivity. Mild symptoms may or may not be provoked by this method. However, allergic symptoms can be reversed by a subcutaneous injection of the neutralising or desensitising dose. The individual would then receive neutralising injections twice a week and would be allowed to eat foods that had been tested. For the multiple-allergic, a combination of neutralising injections for the severe allergies and a rotation diet for the less severe is often the most practical approach.

Many different kinds of tests exist for allergies, one of which is to test the levels of proteins called immunoglobulins in the blood. Traditionally, allergy tests measure the levels of IgE produced when the immune cells are exposed to a particular substance. This immunoglobulin is responsible for classical and immediate allergic reactions. However, more and more scientific attention is being focussed on IgG reactions which are thought to be behind delayed reactions and possibly accounting for the majority of allergies. Tests now exist to measure the quantity of IgG antibodies produced in different foods. These tests may prove to be even more reliable than previous intradermal testing.

Most patients with food allergies also tend to have pyroluria, a stress phenomenon associated with excess pyrroles in the urine which bind vitamin B6 and zinc. Some allergies, such as those associated with wheat, are accompanied by damage to the intestinal mucosa (coeliac disease), resulting in the malabsorption of zinc and/or B6, as well as other nutrients. When the gut wall becomes more leaky this increases the chance of incompletely digested food proteins getting into the blood and causing allergy. Healing the digestive tract is therefore a prerequisite to dealing with allergies.

Reactions to Everyday Drugs

Allergic patients may react adversely when exposed to food dyes, aspirin, foods with salicylates, food additives, food preservatives, and the insecticides used to reduce spoilage of food. Organic food eating is therefore recommended and carefully chosen vendors become most important. Was insecticide used? Were crops sprayed? Was a preservative added? The members of one allergic family were literally driven from their home in Connecticut when the government officials decided to spray the whole landscape to kill the gypsy moths. Air deodorants and perfumes may also be offenders. In air travel one can smell the surge of deodorant wafting through the cabin at regular intervals, to the dismay and discomfort of those allergic to petrochemicals.

The ultimate outcome of careful diagnosis and treatment of the allergic patient with cerebral symptoms may be excellent. The patient must, however, watch for new allergies and follow the carefully prescribed diet and routine of avoidance.

Our Deadly Bread

Hidden sensitivity to one's daily bread may well be the cause of compulsive and ritualistic behaviour, impaired speech development and mood and behaviour changes. Not everyone can digest wheat, rye and other cereal grains. This condition is known as 'coeliac disease', and secondary symptoms may result. In coeliac disease, food may go through the gut undigested. Recent studies have indicated that coeliac disease may be responsible for many cases of 'schizophrenia'. Evidence is accumulating which links various psychiatric disturbances with malabsorption caused by cereal grains, and it is becoming increasingly apparent that for many individuals, daily bread is much less than a blessing.

One of the earliest observations of the relationship between cereal grains and schizophrenia was reported by Dr. Lauretta Bender in 1953, when she noted that schizophrenic children were extraordinarily subject to coeliac disease [21]. By 1966 she had recorded 20 such cases from among more than 2000 schizophrenic children. In 1961 Graff and Handford published data stating that during one year, four out of thirty-seven adult male schizophrenics admitted to the Institute of

Pennsylvania Hospital, Philadelphia, had a history of coeliac disease in childhood 22. These early observations greatly interested Dr. Dohan of the Hospital of the University of Pennsylvania. He noted that these data indicated that 'schizophrenia' occurs far more frequently than chance would predict in children and also in adults with coeliac disease. Dohan believes that an inherited susceptibility to both coeliac disease and 'schizophrenia' may indeed exist and that one may contribute to the development of the other.

The Signs of Wheat-Gluten Sensitivity

The clinical symptoms of coeliac disease and 'schizophrenia' bear marked resemblance. Both physical and psychiatric symptoms are present in children and adults with coeliac disease, although the incidence of 'schizophrenia' is greater in children than in adults. Coeliac disease results in part from an impairment of food absorption from the intestine. Coeliac patients are classically very thin and have a protruding relaxed abdomen. Bowel movements are frequent and are fatty, loose, large and foul. Facial expression is typically shrivelled and drawn, suggesting a state of melancholy. In fact, the psychiatric picture of the coeliac child is not unlike that of the schizophrenic child. Both are dissociated from the world, weepy and introverted. Coeliac patients are also subject to mood disorders such as extreme depression and anxiety. These occur after cereal grain is eaten and subside when such food is carefully avoided. In adults, large blisters may occur on the skin on the back of the hands (dermatitis herpentiformis).

The toxic element high is responsible in coeliac disease is gluten, a protein found in wheat, rye, barley and oats. The mechanisms that produce gluten intolerance have yet to be fully determined. The theory is that intestinal enzymes cannot digest the gluten and accumulating toxic material irritates the lining of the intestinal wall, causing chronic indigestion and malabsorption of all nutrients. Yet another theory suggests that exorphins' found in gluten compete with the body's endorphins which are vital brain chemicals involved in mood. Removal of wheat gluten and similar gluten proteins found in other cereal grains has been shown to improve digestive processes, promote weight gain, and to alleviate mood and psychiatric symptoms.

The importance of considering gluten sensitivity is well

demonstrated in a study by Dr. Dohan in 1969 [23]. He randomly placed all men admitted to a locked psychiatric ward in a Veterans Administration Hospital in Coatsville, Pennsylvania, either on a diet containing no milk or cereals, or on a diet that was relatively high in cereals. All other treatment continued as normal. Midway through the experiment 62% of the group on no milk and cereals were released to a 'full privileges' ward while only 36% of those patients receiving a diet including cereal were able to leave the locked ward. When the wheat gluten was secretly included in the diet, the improved patients relapsed.

The same results were found in a study by Drs Mohan Singh and Stanley Kay, at the Bronx Psychiatric Centre in New York [24]. Fourteen schizophrenics were kept on a gluten-free diet for 12 weeks and given a special drink, containing, among other ingredients, either soy protein for the first four and last four weeks or wheat gluten in the middle four weeks. During the four 'wheat gluten' weeks there was marked deterioration in almost all behavioural yardsticks measured.

These studies indicate that, at present, diet is the crucial factor in treating gluten-sensitive schizophrenics. Therefore, wheat-gluten sensitivity should be considered in the pathogenesis of the 'schizophrenias' and once diagnosis has been made, patients should understand and employ a diet free from milk and cereals.

Recognising wheat-gluten sensitivity is frequently difficult because classical symptoms are often absent. When either the doctor (or nutritionist) or the patient is even vaguely suspicious of gluten sensitivity, a special diet can be undertaken for a trial period. Weeks or months may be required before a marked improvement appears after wheat, rye, barley, oats and milk are removed from the diet. Re-introduction of these grains and milk into the diet usually produces a relapse in months, days or even hours! It is important, then, to maintain a strict adherence to the diet.

With removal of the offending foods, irritability, mood swings, compulsive behaviour and other psychiatric disorders will subside. Dr Dohan suggests that elimination diets should be tried for at least six months to a year. Further investigation is needed to determine how long the milk and cereal free diet must be followed to determine the possibility of developing a 'gluten tolerance' which would permit careful re-introduction of these foods into the diet.

20

AUTISM, LEARNING DIFFICULTIES AND DYSLEXIA

Wendy was 3 years old when her parents realised she was not developing normally. At 48 months her mental age was 21 months. She achieved an IQ of 44 and was classified as retarded. When 4 years old, then testing with an IQ of 49, she began megavitamin therapy. Her attention span went from 10 to 15 seconds to ten minutes. Within three months she began speaking in complete sentences. After six months of treatment her IQ score had jumped to 72. By the age of 8 her IQ score was 85, classifying her as no longer retarded, with low-average ability - a 40 point shift in 4 years.
(Case from by Dr Henry Turkel [1].)

We have known since 1970 that autistic children respond to zinc and B6. Dr Allan Cott from New York was the first to confirm this finding. Dr Catherine Spears, a paediatric neurologist, reported that out of twenty autistic children she was treating, all responded to zinc and B6 [2]. Dr Spears reports that parents, teachers and professionals have all rated the autistic children as improved in both behaviour and speech.

Dr Bernard Rimland of the Institute for Child Behaviour Research in San Diego, California, listened to these reports and tested them on autistic children. The study showed significant improvement in autism when B6 was given. The sixteen patients also had magnesium and vitamin C in adequate supply. Rimland fought with the American Journal of Psychiatry to get it published and finally the article appeared in the April, 1978 issue [2] [3]. Science News [3] Twelve out of sixteen autistic children improved and regressed when the vitamins were swapped for placebos. He found that the addition of magnesium, at half the level of the B6, was even more effective [4].

Magnesium levels are often low in autistic children[5] and the combined supplementation of B6, zinc and magnesium will often lead to improvements. In the decade following Dr Rimland's pioneering study five further studies tested this approach. All reported positive results with the B6 and magnesium combination.

Test for Pyroluria

We have examined and treated children in the age range of 3-15 years who were labelled 'mentally retarded' or 'minimal brain dysfunction' or 'learning disabled'. When the young patient has a high level of pyrroles in the urine, a low serum immunoglobulin A, and facial swelling with a history of frequent colds and middle ear infections, pyroluria should be suspected. The tissue swelling caused by zinc and B6 deficiency prevents the adequate drainage of the auditory tubes from the middle ear to the throat. Immunoglobulin A (IgA) is present in all secretions of the body such as tears, mucus, saliva, breast milk and gastric juices. When IgA is low there is poor resistance and repeated infections may occur.

The Allergy Link

A large percentage of children diagnosed as autistic develop normally until the age of 2 or 3 and then, following repeated ear infections and antibiotic treatment cease developing properly. Autistic children have been found to have an increased number of large food protein fragments in their blood and urine compared to other children [5]. This is an indication of 'leaky gut syndrome' associated with multiply allergies. The extra need for B6 and zinc, both of which are needed to properly digest and use protein, may contribute to incompletely digested proteins getting into the bloodstream. Treatment with antibiotics, which further damage the gut, make the situation worse. As the body increasingly reacts to normal foods as if they were toxins the detoxification systems of the body can get overloaded, allowing harmful biochemicals to disturb brain and nervous system function.

The allergy link has been thoroughly investigated by Dr Rimland from California [6]. He tested the effects of removing wheat, milk or sugar in hundreds of autistic children. About half improved from the removal of any one of these. Wheat and milk are hard to digest and, especially if introduced too early in life, can result in allergy. Sugar is no good for anyone. These foods are definitely worth eliminating.

The Value of Supplements

A large number of studies using nutritional supplements have shown dramatic improvements in IQ and mental performance, especially among dyslexic and other children with learning difficulties, even in Downs Syndrome. When researcher Dr Ruth Harrell heard of a case in which the IQ of a Down's syndrome child went from 20 to 90 points, she decided to explore the ideas that many mentally retarded children might have been born with increased needs for certain vitamins and minerals. In her first study she took 22 mentally retarded children and divided them into two groups. One received vitamin and mineral supplements, the other received placebos (dummy tablets). After four months, the IQ in the group taking the supplements had increased between 5 and 9.6 points; those on placebos showed no change. For the next four months, both groups of children were given the supplements and the average improvement had risen to 10.2 points. Six of the Down's children had improvements of between 10 and 25 IQ points! [7]

The results seemed too good to be true. After all, Down's syndrome is a genetic disease, so how could vitamin supplements increase the intelligence of six of the children so dramatically? This sort of improvement in intelligence would put most of our educationally sub-normal children back in normal classes!

These findings have since been confirmed by three researchers - and contradicted by three more [8]. Why the apparent confusion? Researcher Dr Alex Schauss may have found the answer: it appears that only those children taking thyroid treatment and supplements improved. Neither supplements nor thyroid treatment on their own are expected to help improve intelligence in Down's syndrome patients.

Similar spectacular results have been reported by Dr Henry Turkel in Down's Syndrome, mucopolysaccharidosis and retardation using megavitamin therapy [1,9,10]. He was able to show major physical, skeletal and intellectual normalising over years of nutritional treatment. One retarded child went from an IQ of 48 to 85 over a four year period.

Many Down's Syndrome children had spectacular physical changes over a decade of treatment.

Earlier work in nutrition, such as a study by Kubula in 1960, [11] had shown that increased vitamin status was associated with increased intelligence. He divided 351 students into high and low vitamin C groups, depending on the levels in their blood. The students' IQ was then measured and found to average 113 and 109 respectively: those with higher levels of vitamin C had an average of 4.5 IQ points more.

The less refined foods you eat the cleverer you are, concluded some researchers at the Massachusetts Institute for Technology. They found that the higher the proportion of refined carbohydrates in the diet, the lower the IQ score. The difference was almost 25 points! [12]

Great improvement in intelligence has also been shown with autistic children, and those with learning difficulties. In a study by Dr Colgan on 16 children with learning and behavioural difficulties, each child had his or her individual nutrient needs determined [13]. Half the children were then given supplements, while the others acted as a control. Each child attended a remedial reading course designed to improve reading age by one year. Over the next 22 weeks teachers carefully monitored the reading age, IQ and behaviour of the children.

Those not taking supplements showed an average increase in IQ of 8.4 points and in reading age of 1.1 years. However, the group on supplements had an improvement in IQ of 17.9 points and their reading age went up by 1.8 years. The most likely explanation, Dr Colgan concluded, was the decline in toxic levels of metals like lead, which are known to have detrimental effects on intelligence.

Brain Pollution

A number of other studies have proved the connection between lead levels and intelligence. One researcher, Dr Needleman, [14] who has tested thousands of children, has not yet found a single child with high lead who has an IQ above 125. Normally 5 per cent of the population fall above this measurement. Since the advent of lead-free petrol blood lead levels are fortunately dropping. Copper is another toxic element that has been reported to be high in dyslexic children [15]. Since zinc and vitamin C are both antagonists of copper this is another possible explanation for their often reported benefit.

21

THE ATTENTION DEFICIT DISASTER

Stephen, aged 6, had a history of hyperactivity, with severely disturbed sleep and disruptive behaviour at home and at school. Threatened with expulsion from school because of his impossible behaviour, his parents were given two weeks to improve matters. They contacted the Hyperactive Childrens Support Group and evening primrose oil was suggested. A dose of 1.5g was rubbed into the skin morning and evening. The school was unaware of this, but after five days the teacher telephoned the mother to say that never in 30 years of teaching had she seen such a dramatic change in a child's behaviour. After three weeks the evening primrose oil was stopped, and one week later the school again complained. The oil was then introduced with good effect.
(Case gratefully supplied from the HACSG records.)

The child can't sit still, can't concentrate for more than a few minutes, is volatile, gets into fights and disrupts the class. This is the teacher's nightmare, and more and more there's one or more such child in every class. These are classic signs of an ever-increasing syndrome known as ADHD - attention deficit hyperactivity disorder, sometimes abbreviated to ADD or hyperactivity. Often, but not always linked to dyslexia, these children have a hard time at school and at home, performing badly, getting into trouble and are often shunted from school to school. Substantial evidence is linking the decline in school standards and increase in delinquency to an epidemic of hyperactivity, now known as ADD - attention deficit disorder, which affects one in ten boys in the UK.

Can Hyperactivity lead to Delinquency?
As teenagers they are more likely to become young offenders and develop chemical dependency. Angela Devlin, a teacher with 25 years

Is Your Child Hyperactive?

Do these characteristics apply?

Overactive	Doesn't Finish Projects
Fidgets	Can't Sit Still At Meals
Doesn't Stay With Games	Wears Out Toys, Furniture, etc.
Talks Too Much	Doesn't Follow Directions
Clumsy	Fights With Other Children
Unpredictable	Teases
Doesn't Respond To Discipline	Gets Into Things
Speech Problem	Temper Tantrums
Doesn't Listen To Whole Story	Defiant
Hard To Get To Bed	Irritable
Reckless	Unpopular With Peers
Impatient	Lies
Accident Prone	Bed wetter
Destructive	

Score 5 if a symptom is severe, 3 if moderate and 1 if not present. A score below 45 is normal. Higher scores indicate your child may benefit from the following:

- Eliminate chemical additives and sugar
- Test and eliminate allergens (often wheat, dairy or eggs)
- Supplement essential fatty acids (both $\Omega 3$ and $\Omega 6$)
- Supplement vitamin B3, B6, magnesium, zinc and other key nutrients
- Test for and detoxify toxic elements

experience dealing with children with special needs, examined the link between educational failure and future offending behaviour in her book Criminal Classes - Offenders at School (Waterside Press, 1995)[1]. She found that a high proportion of young offenders were dyslexic and hyperactive and ended up being punished and failing with little opportunity to build self-esteem. In a study of 82 chemically-dependent patients of Turning Point, an alcohol and drug rehabilitation centre, Dr Morton and Hardman found 98% also had dyslexia and/or ADD [2]. A ten year follow-up of 64 adolescents, diagnosed as hyperactive as children, found 25% were still engaging in anti-social or delinquent behaviour [3].

Of course, the critical question is what is causing this epidemic of ADD? Is it the result of poor parenting, poor schooling, poor diet or inheritance? Certainly, if the problem isn't recognised, the child won't receive the special attention needed both at school and at home. Yet, few children are being evaluated for chemical, nutritional or allergic factors. The main treatment given to millions of school children classified with ADD is drugs. One drug alone, Ritalin, is prescribed to over 1 million children each year in the US alone [4].

Acquired or Inherited?

Some researchers blame heredity. Dr Russell Barkley, of the University of Massachusetts, reports that nearly half ADD children have a parent of sibling with the disorder. Dr James Swanson, a psychologist from the University of California, believes that something may go wrong in pregnancy, perhaps due to fetal distress possibly brought on by anti-nutrients such as lead or alcohol. Dr Lawrence Greenberg, an ADD specialist from Minnesota, estimates that a quarter of surviving premature infants have ADD. Drs Hardman and Morton also found, from taking family histories, an extremely high percentage of family members having a history of diseases associated with altered biochemistry, immune or metabolic deficiencies. In the case of the patients themselves, 82% had allergic or immunological problems which had manifested before going to school, yet had rarely been treated. ADD is also much more likely to occur in boys than girls, affecting about 4 boys for every 1 girl. Irene Colquhoun and Sally Bunday, who founded and run the Hyperactive Children's Support Group (see Useful Addresses on page 200), also found a preponderance of fair and ginger-haired children among those with ADD. Dyslexia is also often familial and has been linked with genetic transmission associated with chromosome 15. Research is currently going on to examine the link between immune disorders, dyslexia and left-handedness. Current theories are that there is often an inherited imbalance which makes the child prone to allergic, immunological, or metabolic disorders.

Brain Fat Deficiency?

One of these metabolic disorders may concern the ability to convert essential fats into vital brain chemicals. Bunday and Colquhoun first reported the link in 1981 having noticed that abnormal thirst is a common characteristic of ADD children. Another is dry skin. Eczema and asthma are also commonly found. Each of these symptoms are associated with 'prostaglandin' imbalance, chemical modulators that affect the brain, inflammatory reactions and water balance. Prostaglandins are made directly from essential fats found in the diet, and are then converted by enzymes, dependent on certain vitamins and minerals. Bunday and Colquhoun theorised that ADD children may be deficient in essential fatty acids either because their need is higher or because they absorb them poorly or they don't convert them well into prostaglandins [5]. They went on to test the effects of evening primrose oil, a rich source of gamma-linolenic acid, on some of the children.

Stephen, a six year-old with a history of hyperactivity, disturbed sleep and disruptive behaviour, was one of them. He had been threatened with expulsion and his parents had been given two weeks to improve matters. He was given three capsules of evening primrose oil (1.5g), with the oil rubbed into his skin morning and evening. The school was unaware of this but after five days the teacher telephoned the mother and said that never in 30 years teaching had she seen such a dramatic change in a child's behaviour. After three weeks the evening primrose oil was stopped and one week later the school complained. The oil was then reintroduced with good effect.

However, anecdotal reports don't carry much weight and it wasn't until last year that researchers at Purdue University in the US found altered fatty acid metabolism and lowered levels of these essential substances in the blood of children diagnosed with ADHD, compared to controls [6]. Two controlled studies have been performed since Colquhoun and Bunday's report, however neither produced significant behavioural changes. No studies have yet been published on the effects of fish oils, rich in DHA, a fatty acid essential to brain function. Children with low DHA levels have been shown to have poor mental performance later in life. Controversially, Coca-Cola is launching a drink aimed at the adolescent market which, it is claimed, will promote learning ability due to the addition of DHA.

The Vitamin Connection

Essential fats have to be converted into prostaglandins by two enzymes which depend on the presence of vitamin B3 (niacin), B6, C, biotin, zinc and magnesium (see chart). The possibility of a connection between B3 and B6 deficiency and ADD has been investigated. One of the best reported results was a controlled study by Dr Abram Hoffer, who gave large amounts of vitamin C (3g) and B3 (niacinamide 1.5g or more). Only one of the 33 children in the trial failed to respond [7]. Other studies have shown improvement with B3 and B6 supplementation specifically when the child has low serotonin levels, an important brain neurotransmitter. Some children may be zinc or magnesium deficient, both of which can produce symptoms associated with ADD. The symptoms of magnesium deficiency, for example, are excessive fidgeting, anxious restlessness, coordination problems and learning difficulties in the presence of a normal IQ. Although it is unlikely, on the basis of the studies to date, that ADD is purely a nutrient deficiency disease, some children are deficient and do respond very well.

Brain Pollution

As well as investigating nutrient levels, anti-nutrients can induce ADD symptoms. Top of the toxins is lead which produces symptoms of aggression, poor impulse control and attention span. Another is excess copper, which has been reported to occur in some ADD children. One study found a link between high aluminium and hyperactivity. Many toxic elements deplete the body of essential nutrients. Lead and copper deplete zinc levels and may contribute to deficiency. So too does tartrazine, a common food additive added to children's drinks. Dr Neil Ward, from the University of Surrey, found that adding tartrazine to drinks increased the amount of zinc excreted in the urine, perhaps by binding to zinc in the blood and preventing it from being used by the body [8]. In this study they also found emotional and behavioural changes in every child who drank the drink containing tartrazine. Four out of the ten children in the study had severe reactions, three developing eczema or asthma within 45 minutes of ingestion.

The Allergy Link

Tartrazine is one of many chemical additives known to provoke allergic reactions that bring on symptoms of ADD. Over 200,000 tonnes of chemical additives are added to food each year, or approximately 10lbs per person. Some children aren't coping well with this level of chemical onslaught.

As long ago as 1975 Dr Ben Feingold reported successful treatment of ADD by eliminating chemical additives and foods containing salicylates such as many herbs, spices, nuts, berries, coffee, tea and certain other foods and drinks. His controversial Feingold diet has been studied extensively and produced reasonable results, especially in relation to the elimination of chemical additives. Other substances often found to induce behavioural changes are wheat, dairy produce, eggs and sugar. Reactions to sugar are, in many cases, not due to allergy as such but a craving brought on by low blood sugar levels. Dr Schoenthaler and his team found a clear correlation between sugar/junk food intake and anti-social behaviour. By reducing sugar intake alone halved disciplinary actions in incarcerated juvenile offenders.

Probably of all the avenues so far researched the link between hyperactivity and allergy is the most established and worthy of pursuit in any child showing signs of this syndrome. Associated symptoms that are strongly linked to allergy include nasal problems and excessive mucus, ear infections, facial swelling and discolouration around the eyes, tonsillitis, digestive problems, bad breath, eczema, asthma, headaches and bed-wetting. Significant advances have been made in allergy testing and, in the long-run it is worth having a proper allergy test using the quantitative IgG ELISA method. These tests can identify foods that an individual reacts to from a single blood sample and usually cost between £150 and £300 depending on the number of foods tested and the chosen laboratory.

Conventional Treatment vs the Optimum Nutrition Approach

The optimum nutrition approach to ADD involves a combination of these discussed factors. Most practitioners using this approach to ADD have reported significant improvement in at least two thirds of children. This is substantially better than any drugs currently prescribed for ADD. Ritalin, the most frequently prescribed, helps about a third of children and makes a third worse.

Dr Bernard Rimland studied the effect of the nutrient approach to ADD on 191 children. Dr Humphrey Osmond decided to compare this to the reported results with drugs. He reported the total number taking each drug, the number helped, the number worsened and the 'relative efficacy ratio' (see chart below). This is the number helped divided by the number worsened. So if twice as many are helped as worsened, the ratio is 2. If the same number of people are helped as worsened then the ratio is 1. The results showed that as many ADD sufferers are worsened by medication as are helped, with Mellaril being the best drug. In stark contrast 18 times as many sufferers are helped with nutrients, with 66% responding to this approach.

The skillful application of all the factors discussed in this article by a nutrition consultant may increase both the success rate and degree of improvement.

Vitamins vs Drugs - Which Work Best?

Medication	Total	No. Helped	No. Worsened	Relative Efficacy Ratio
Dexedrine	172	44	80	0.55
Ritalin	66	22	27	0.81
Mysoline	10	4	4	1.00
Valium	106	31	31	1.00
Dilantin	204	57	43	1.33
Benadril	151	34	25	1.36
Stelazine	120	40	28	1.43
Deanol	73	17	10	1.70
Mellaril	277	101	55	1.84
All drugs	**1591**	**440**	**425**	**1.00**
Vitamins	**191**	**127**	**7**	**18.14**

22

CRIME- NOURISHMENT OR PUNISHMENT?

Anne was notorious for her anti-authoritarian attitudes and violence. She had lived in care since the age of 10, and had a history of assault and burglary, and bouts of severe depression and solvent abuse. Analyses showed abnormal glucose tolerance, zinc, magnesium and B vitamin deficiencies. Here energy level was very low in the morning and she'd often have drops in energy during the day, leaving her depressed and edgy. Within three weeks on a low-sugar diet plus supplements she had freed herself of drugs, was no longer depressed, had improved energy and described how she had never felt so relaxed. She continued to improve and gradually, frowns gave way to smiles.

When someone commits a crime what do you do? Punish them as a means of deterrent; remove them from society to prevent further crime; or try to understand the causes of deviant behaviour in order to socially rehabilitate the offender? In the world of rehabilitation one factor that is completely overlooked is nutrition. Bernard Gesch, a former probation officer, and now director of Natural Justice, a charity based in Cumbria, believes that the criminal justice system falsely places all the emphasis on social issues, ignoring physical factors such as nutrition. "There are many chemicals around us that are known to affect behaviour. Our environment is increasingly polluted. Our food supply has fundamentally changed. In the same way that we don't notice ageing, how would we notice the effects of gradual changes to our diet and environment?" says Gesch, yet the effects are there.

The fact is that all thoughts and consequently behaviour are processed through the brain and nervous system which is totally dependent on nutrition. Approximately half of all the glucose in the

Diet Behaviour Record for Anne (Self rating)

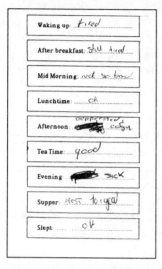
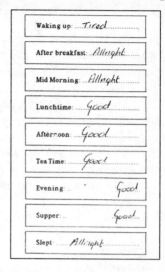

Waking up: tired
After breakfast: still tired
Mid Morning: not so bad
Lunchtime: ok
Afternoon: ~~depressed~~ edgy
Tea Time: good
Evening: ~~~~ sick
Supper: less to you
Slept: ok

Waking up: Tired
After breakfast: Allright
Mid Morning: Allright
Lunchtime: good
Afternoon: Good
Tea Time: Good
Evening: Good
Supper: Good
Slept: Allright

BEFORE: 3rd November   **AFTER:** 22nd November

blood goes to power the brain which is also dependent on a second by second supply of micro-nutrients - vitamins, minerals and essential fatty acids. Anti-nutrients such as lead and cadmium fundamentally affect brain function. "What we're trying to do" says Gesch "is introduce something new into the criminal justice system, that is the existence of the human brain." His research, and others, has identified biochemical factors that influence behaviour: exposure to neurotoxins; nutrient deficiencies; paradoxical reactions to given substances; and reactive hypoglycaemia.

Reactive Hypoglycaemia

In a remarkable pilot project, known as SCASO (South Cumbria Alternative Sentencing Options) young offenders were required, as part of their sentence, to undergo 'nutritional rehabilitation'. The participants underwent a series of tests for vitamin and mineral levels, toxic minerals, blood sugar balance, as well as dietary assessment. "The most common problems were glucose intolerance and zinc deficiency.

Every single person we tested had abnormal glucose tolerance on a five hour glucose tolerance test." says Gesch 1. The importance of glucose control in relation to behaviour is a consistent finding in the criminal population. In Finland Virkkunen investigated 69 habitual offenders for glucose balance. Every single one had reactive hypoglycaemia. A later study confirmed higher insulin activity during glucose tolerance tests among habitually violent offenders 2.

In the US Professor Stephen Schoenthaler, head of the Department of Sociology and Criminal Justice at California State University, has reported a 21% reduction in anti-social behaviour, a 25% reduction in assaults, a 75% reduction in the use of restraints, and a 100% reduction in suicides when 3,000 inmates were placed on an experimental diet which reduced refined and sugary foods 3. These results were confirmed in a double-blind study involving 1,382 detained juvenile offenders placed on a reduced sugar diet. There was a 44% reduction in antisocial behaviour with most significant reductions among the serious offenders 4.

The rebound 'low', known as reactive hypoglycemia, after a rapid increase in blood sugar levels, induced by sugar, sweets or stimulants, known as reactive hypoglycemia, and is associated with extreme tiredness, depression, aggression and attempted suicide. According to Gesch "Of the 40 to 50 people we worked with on SCASO we could create an effect within a week or two."

Brain Pollution

One of the most invisible effects on behaviour is that of unseen pollution. A worldwide consensus of research has shown that high lead levels equates to low intellectual performance and anti-social behaviour. The correlation between high lead and increased anti-social or delinquent behaviour was found in an observational study of 1,000 children by Freeman and co-workers in New South Wales 5, by Needleman and co-workers in the US who found anti-social behaviour correlated to high dentine lead levels in 2,146 children 6 and by Thomson and co-workers in Edinburgh who found deviant behaviour correlated with high blood lead levels 7. Pihl and Ervin found a correlation between high hair lead and cadmium in violent inmates compared to non-violent inmates 8. Other researchers have confirmed an association between high lead and cadmium and deviant behaviour.

The levels of neurotoxins, like lead and cadmium, that produces an effect on behaviour is around 1% of the level needed to produce physical symptoms, which indicates how sensitive that part of the brain involved with socialisation is to environmental and nutritional changes.

Nutrients Against Crime

Supplementing zinc, which is an antagonist of these heavy metals, has had favourable effects on behaviour. Researcher Alex Schauss found significantly higher levels of lead, cadmium and copper in violent, anti-social adults compared to non-offenders [9]. The effect of zinc on brain function is consistent with previous studies that have linked zinc deficiency to hyperactivity, learning and eating disorders.

Needless to say, nutritional deficiency is rife among young offenders. Professor Schoenthaler found evidence of widespread folic acid, thiamine (vitamin B1) and vitamin C deficiencies. Even adding orange juice to the diets of detainees, which contains each of these nutrients, produced a staggering 47% reduction in anti-social behaviour among juvenile offenders [10].

Deficiencies in calcium, magnesium, zinc, selenium and essential fatty acids have also been shown to correlate with increases in violence. The simple addition of a multivitamin and mineral supplement containing RDA levels of nutrients has been shown to have extremely positive effects on behaviour in US prison populations, according to recent research by Schoenthaler, who is coming to Britain in April to present his latest findings.

Anti-Social Foods

The fourth factor proving to be significant is that of paradoxical reactions to foods. Severe allergic reactions can produce Jekyll & Hyde changes in behaviour as has been well reported in hyperactive children with chemical or food intolerances [11]. Menzies found that, in a study of 25 children with tension fatigue syndrome, all had disturbed sleep, 84% had abnormal EEG and 72% had digestive problems. All consumed a diet unusually high in refined foods and chemical additives [12].

Of the few studies so far conducted all shows dramatic reductions in re-offending among offenders maintained on low-sugar, high nutrient diets. According to Gesch "75 per cent of our referrals were for violent offences, many of whom were multiple offenders. Of those kept of the combined social and nutritional regime none re-offended with a violent offence by the end of the eighteen-month pilot study."[13] The treatment provided, namely supplements, cost between £4 and £10 a month, compared to the average cost of £2,000 a month to keep someone in prison.

Other Factors

As well as these factors there are at least seven biochemical imbalances which can result in violent behaviour. These are, in their probable order of importance, the following:

1   Pyroluria (combined zinc and B6 deficiency).
2   Histadelia - high histamine levels in the blood. (This characterises the addictive person).
3   Excess copper (or other metals) and histapenia.
4   Increased testosterone can lead to rape. Treated with progesterone injections.
5   Psychomotor epilepsy attacks (cerebellar stimulation helps).
6   XYY Syndrome - excessive height and violence in males.
7   Premenstrual syndrome (PMS), coupled with zinc, magnesium and vitamin B6 deficiency.

Most of these biotypes can easily be diagnosed and nutritionally treated. The stumbling block at present is the lack of trained personnel and a laboratory to perform the tests accurately.

Who's to Blame?

The crux of the issue in criminal justice is culpability. If behaviour is thought of purely as a psychological/social phenomena then the blame rests on the individual and their relationship with society. Hence the current strategy of punishment, removal from society, and social rehabilitation. If brain function, and all the factors that affect brain function, is put into the equation then issues around nutrition and environmental pollution have to be considered.

This will necessitate the establishment of diagnostic centres at each prison and hospital. Education is so often the key, and the establishment of prison nutrition clubs to promote awareness of good nutrition among patients, prisoners and security personnel, backed up by the availability of food charts and literature, would do much to improve the awareness so sadly lacking. Perhaps even more pressing than the need for further research into schizophrenia is the need for a research institute dealing with psychopathic, violent or anti-social behaviour. The good news is that more and more research is being carried out in the US and in the UK to support the very positive results already achieved.

23

BEATING ADDICTIONS

Chris, who became addicted to heroine, was taken off heroine and given prescriptions for Methadone, Temazepan, Diazepan and Valium (check spelling), to which he became addicted. He then tried a nutrition based detox programme called Narconon, which includes a 'purification phase' involving large amounts of niacin and other nutrients, plus daily saunas. "It's the easiest detox I've ever done.Having gone through the purification I understand why, after previous detox's, I was still craving. In the beginning of the sauna programme I would get flashbacks, but after two weeks I was feeling full of energy, and happy which has stayed with me since I finished. I'm keeping on the vitamins. I've closed that chapter of my life without a doubt." Jim spent 12 years addicted to heroine and methadone and couldn't quit. "This is the only programme that has worked for me. I've been off drugs for 5 months. Here withdrawal was not nearly as bad as I thought it would be. The vitamins must have helped. My body has totally changed. Now I feel totally new. For me there's no going back to all that." (Cases from Narconon clients)

In the words of one of the founders of optimum nutrition, Dr Roger Williams, "No one who follows good nutrition practice will ever become alcoholic." Addiction, whether it be to alcohol or heroine, doesn't happen overnight. On average, it takes seven years of hard drinking before addiction is likely to set in. Those who are well nourished are unlikely to become addicted, or to be so attracted to addictive substances, most of which create a lift in energy, sought by the undernourished.

Of course addiction is not only chemical, it is psychological and psychological factors, as well as drug abuse, are usually present in those who become addicted. Obviously, psychological factors that predispose a person to addiction will need to be dealt with alongside

Are You Addicted?

Do you consider yourself dependent, or have a regular intake of an addictive substance and some of the following symptoms?

Depression or feelings of doom
Nervousness and anxiety
Craving for sweets or alcohol
Irritability or rages,
Headaches
Weight problems (either way)
Extreme tiredness or weakness
Dizziness or feeling faint
Morning nausea
Blurred vision
Transient muscle aches or joint pain
Insomnia and nightmares

If a majority of these apply you may benefit from:
• A high strength B Complex giving 100mg of most B's
• Niacin 500mg to 1,000mg, am and pm
• Pantothenic acid (B5) 500mg, am and pm
• Vitamin B6 100mg, am Folic acid 1 to 2mg, am
• Vitamin C 10 grams a day spread throughout the day
• L-glutamine powder, 5 grams am and pm
• plus enough essential fats including GLA and minerals including calcium, magnesium, potassium and zinc

The best diet is highly alkaline forming, meaning high in fresh fruit and vegetables, and rich in complex or slow-releasing carbohydrates and free from sugar and stimulants.

nutrition intervention. However, whatever the cause, once a person is addicted, this has chemical and physiological effects. You can't just remove the addictive substance without inducing withdrawal symptoms, sometimes severe enough to cause death.

In the Genes?

There is supporting evidence for a genetic factor in some people, predisposing them to addiction. A large proportion of addictive types are histadelic. This runs through the family so history of addiction, depression, suicide and mental illness of a compulsive/obsessive nature, is a good clue to histamine playing a part. The solution is to follow the advice given in Chapter 14.

Empty Calories Lead to Addiction

One study with mice gives a clue to another predisposing factor. The mice in this study were split into two groups: one given a healthy diet; the other a junk food diet. Both had free access to water or alcohol. The junk food mice soon became alcoholic and died prematurely. The health food mice stayed teetotal and lived to a ripe, old age.

As the alcoholic mice become more and more nutrient deficient, they became less interested in food, more interested in alcohol. Alcohol not only stops you absorbing. It also effects appetite. So bad nutrition not only leads to alcoholism, but alcoholism leads to bad nutrition. It's a vicious downhill spiral. The same link between junk food and addiction has also been recorded in humans [1].

The Sugar Connection

Most alcoholics and drug addicts have hypoglycemia. One way of raising your blood sugar level is to smoke a cigarette, have a coffee, chocolate, alcohol or take a drug, from cannabis to cocaine. A group of researchers in 1973 decided to test how many of 200 alcoholics had abnormal blood sugar balance with a glucose tolerance test. No less than 97% came up positive [2].

Many people control their blood sugar level by eating, drinking and smoking substances that alter their body chemistry. There's also a synergy of these pharmacological agents in food and drink. Patricia Much found that high coffee consumption could precipitate alcoholism, because the shakiness from coffee can be controlled by alcohol [3].

Allergy or Addiction?

Addictions have a lot in common with 'hidden' allergies. Often the allergic substance becomes addictive, and if it isn't consumed, withdrawal symptoms set in which can be relieved by consuming the allergen. This is why people often feel worse on a short fast, until the withdrawal phase is over, and then they feel much better.

Addicts also test allergic to their addictive substance. Drs Philpott and Kalita found that 75% of tobacco smokers tested allergic to tobacco on skin tests [4]. In our allergy clinic we find the percentage is even higher. Most allergies require a 5 to 10 day avoidance before a person becomes symptom free. A similar length of time is often required for addictions.

Alcohol Addiction

Pronounced nutritional deficiency states are well recorded in many drug addictions.

In alcoholics common deficiencies are for vitamin B1, zinc and protein. These deficiencies, in turn, bring on mental illness even in the absence of alcohol, as illustrated by the story of one 61 year old woman from New Zealand, diagnosed with schizophrenia [5]. She refused medication for four months, had the delusion she was dying from cancer, and neglected her nutrition. She was admitted to hospital and went into a coma. She was given thiamine, vitamin B1, and responded in three hours. As well as inducing deficiencies alcohol reduces appetite and impairs absorption. When there is organic damage such as pancreatitis, cirrhosis or hepatitis, appetite is further impaired.

The first step in treating addiction is a prepare the person for withdrawal by correcting these deficiencies. A number of researchers have found that megadoses of a cocktail of nutrients, given orally as supplements or intravenously, can virtually eliminate symptoms of withdrawal. Key nutrients are vitamins B1,B2, B3, B6, B12, folic acid, zinc, and selenium, plus amino acids, fatty acids and electrolytic minerals, including sodium, potassium, calcium and magnesium. In some surveys 40% of alcoholics have been found to have folic acid anaemia [6]. Alcohol also blocks the body's ability to make use of essential fatty acids. According to recent studies supplementing GLA reduces cravings and side effects.

In 1974 Dr Russel Smith in the US gave 507 hard-core alcoholics 3-5 grams on niacin/vitamin C a day for a year [7]. At the end of the year 71% were sober. Dr Hoffer and Osmond have reported a 75% success rate after a year, compared to 30% success on counselling using niacin, B6 and C [8]. B6 deficiency may account for some of the perceptual distortions that occur in alcohol intoxication and withdrawal.

Another useful nutrient is the amino acid l-glutamine [9]. Dr William Shive showed that glutamine has a protective effect against alcohol and protects bacteria from alcohol poisoning. If given to rats it decreases voluntary alcohol consumption. The ideal intake is 5 to 10 grams a day.

Heroine and Methadone addiction

Dr Alfred Libby and Irwin Stone pioneered mega-doses of vitamin C in detoxifying addicts [10]. In one study involving 30 heroine addicts they gave 30 to 85 grams a day and achieved a 100% success rate [11]. In 1972 Pawlek also had good results using 3 grams of vitamin C and niacin [12].

Both heroine addiction and alcoholism increases acid levels in the body, causing a depletion of calcium and potassium. In 1973 Dr Blackman decided to test what would happen if he neutralised the acidity [13]. He gave 19 heroine addicts sodium and potassium bicarbonate, plus calcium carbonate every half hour for two hours, followed by a two hour break, repeating the cycle until withdrawal was over. All volunteers said the symptoms were either completely eliminated or considerably reduced. 16 out of 19 reported no severe symptoms. Of the others, symptoms lasted for no more than 4 hours.

Nicotine Addiction

One of the most common, and socially acceptable addictions is to nicotine in tobacco. The same principles apply here as with other addictions. An alkaline diet or the use of alkaline salts certainly helps reduce craving, as does megadoses of vitamin C and niacin, among other nutrients. Most smokers are hypoglycemic so a diet with slow-releasing carbohydrates, no sugar, tea and coffee is essential. Extra chromium, B6 and zinc also help to stabilise blood sugar. These nutritional factors, plus counselling to deal with the psychological and behavioural factors, plus gradual reduction of nicotine intake are highly effective for those who wish to quit.

Tranquilliser Addiction

A quarter of a million people in the UK are addicted to tranquillisers. It is ironic that these are the very drugs often given to heroine or methadone addicts. One again, the same principles apply, building up a sugar and stimulant free diet, with the back-up of supplements and counselling, provides the best opportunity for becoming drug-free.

Why Withdrawal and Detoxification are Different

One consistent, and yet widely ignored finding is that withdrawal from a drug doesn't mean the person is decontaminated [14]. Most drugs take months to completely leave the system, with residues stored in body cells. Hence, high level nutritional support in the months following withdrawal is vital for long-term success, until the addict is truly 'clean'. This approach has been incorporated into the highly successful Narconon programme (see Useful Addresses on page 200), a new approach to rehabilitating drug and alcohol users, based on optimum nutrition principles. Narconon claims more than a 70% success rate after two years. Among its supporters are Kirstie Alley, star of Cheers, formerly an alcohol and cocaine addict.

The Narconon programme consists of three stages, usually lasting three months, carried out in a residential centre with full supervision. The first stage is withdrawal when users are taken off all drugs including prescribed drugs. Instead they are given a special vitamins and minerals six times a day, and, in some cases, intravenous vitamins. This is backed up with a special calcium and magnesium drink, Cal-Mag, which virtually eliminates the terrible cramping and nerve pain associated with opiate withdrawal. The nutrient regime is backed up by 24 hour counselling support. Purification, the second stage, involves a combination of niacin (B3), saunas and exercise aimed to sweat out drug residues that can remain in the body for months. Niacin, is gradually increased up to 2,000mg a day, followed by exercise and four hours in the sauna, drinking a lot of purified water.

In conclusion, some highly successful strategies for dealing with addiction have been tested and proven to work. Sadly, very few addiction treatment centres apply these strategies and consequently have poor success rates. Many ignore biochemical aspects of addiction and simply involve withdrawal and counselling. A radical rethink on the treatment of addiction is badly needed.

24

EATING DISORDERS AND ANOREXIA

One of the greatest shortcomings of human logic is the unquestioned belief that psychological problems, be it of behaviour or intelligence, are influenced only by psychological factors, and that physiological problems are influenced only by physiological factors. This presupposes that mind and body are separate, that the energy of mind and of body are two different things. Our experience contradicts this. Alcohol alters your state of mind. Psychological stress makes muscles tense. Ask a chemist, an anatomist and a psychologist to define where the mind starts and the body ends and they will find that the two are intimately interconnected. The same is especially true of anorexia because it is a behavioural disorder involving eating, a physiological event.

Anorexia was first identified by Dr William Gull in 1874. He advocated "The patient should be fed at regular intervals, and surrounded by persons who could have moral control over them, relations and friends being generally the worst attendants." Today, treatment is often essentially the same, summed up as "drug them, feed them and let them get on with their lives" in an article in the Guardian describing treatment in 'leading hospitals'. The 'modern' approach includes 'behaviour therapy' i.e. rewards and privileges, and drugs to induce compliance. The drugs include psychotropic drugs such as chlorpromazine, sedatives and anti-depressants. The diet is high carbohydrate, sometimes as much as 5,000 kcals, with little regard to quality.

The idea that nutrition, or malnutrition could play a part in the development and treatment of this condition did not really emerge until the 1980s when scientists began to realise just how similar the symptoms and risk factors of anorexia and zinc deficiency were (see table overleaf). As early as 1973 two zinc researchers, Hambidge and Silverman, concluded that, "whenever there is appetite loss in children zinc deficiency should be suspected". In 1979, Bakan, a Canadian health researcher noticed that the symptoms of anorexia and zinc deficiency were similar in a number of respects and proposed that clinical trials be undertaken to test its effectiveness in treatment. Meanwhile, David Horrobin, most renowned for his research into evening primrose oil, proposed that "anorexia nervosa is due to a combined deficiency of zinc and EFA's."

Zinc Hypothesis Confirmed

In 1980 the first trial started at the University of Kentucky. The researchers discovered that 10 out 13 patients admitted with anorexia and 8 out of 14 patients with bulimia were zinc deficient on admission. After vigourous refeeding they became even more zinc deficient. Since zinc is required to digest and utilise protein, from which body tissue is made, they recommended that extra zinc, above that required to correct deficiency, should be given as the anorexic starts to eat and gain weight.

In 1984 the penny dropped with two important research findings and the first case of an anorexic treated with zinc. The first study showed that animals deprived on zinc very rapidly developed loss of appetite, and that if these animals were force fed a zinc deficient diet to gain weight they became seriously ill. The second study showed that zinc deficiency damages the intestinal wall and therefore the absorption of nutrients including zinc, potentially leading to a vicious spiral of deficiency.

Then, in August 1984 Professor Bryce-Smith, renowned for his exposure of the dangers of lead, and Dr. Simpson, a doctor from Reading, reported the first case of anorexia treated with zinc. The patient was a thirteen year-old girl, tearful and depressed, weighing 37kg. She was referred to a consultant psychiatrist but, despite counselling, three months later her weight was 31.5 kg (under 5 stone). Within two months of zinc supplementation at a level of 45mg per day her weight returned to 44.5 kg, she was cheerful again, and tests for zinc deficiency were normal.

Scientists all over the world started to test the effects of zinc on anorexia. Two Swedish doctors at the University of Goteburg reported that "our initial patient is currently maintained on zinc supplementation (45mg p.d.). She is doing very well: her weight as well as her menstruations are normalised." Meanwhile, the first double-blind trial with 15 anorexics was being carried out at the University of California. In 1987 the researchers reported their findings: "Zinc supplementation was followed by a decrease in depression and anxiety. Our data suggest that individuals with anorexia nervosa may be at risk of zinc deficiency and may respond favourably after zinc supplementation." By 1990 many researchers had found that over half anorexic patients showed clear biochemical evidence of zinc deficiency. In 1994 Dr Birmingham and colleagues carried out a double-blind controlled trial giving 100mg of zinc gluconate. They concluded that " the rate of increase in body mass of the zinc supplemented group was twice that of the placebo group and this difference was statistically significant." Sadly, many treatment centres still fail to supplement those suffering from anorexia with zinc.

Mind or Body?

The fact that high levels of zinc supplementation help to treat anorexia does not mean the cause of anorexia is zinc deficiency. Psychological issues may, and probably do, bring about change in the eating habits of susceptible people. By avoiding eating a young girl can repress the signs of growing up. Menstruation stops, breast size decreases and the body stays small. Starvation induces a kind of 'high' by stimulating changes in important brain chemicals, that may help to block out difficult feelings and issues that are too hard to face. But once the route of not eating is chosen and becomes established zinc deficiency is almost inevitable both due to poor intake and poor absorption. With it comes a further loss of appetite and even more depression, disperceptions, and the inability to cope with the stresses that face many adolescents, especially girls, growing up in the 1990s.

The optimum nutrition approach to help someone with anorexia, or bulimia, is best carried alongside work with a skilled psychotherapist. The nutritional approach emphasizes quality of food rather than quantity, including supplements to ensure vitamin and mineral sufficiency, and of course 45mg of elemental zinc per day, halving the level once weight gain is achieved and maintained.

Anorexia		Zinc
	Symptoms	
Weight loss		Weight loss
Loss of appetite		Loss of appetite
Amenorrhoea		Amenorrhoea
Impotence in males		Impotence in males
Nausea		Nausea
Skin lesions		Skin lesions
Malabsorption		Malabsorption
Disperceptions		Disperceptions
Depression		Depression
Anxiety		Anxiety
	Risk factors	
Female under 25		Female under 25
Stress		Stress
Puberty		Puberty

The Amino Acid Connection

Loss of weight and loss of muscle tissue is an indication of protein deficiency. This can be the result of either insufficient intake, or inadequate digestion, absorption, or metabolism. The amino acids valine, isoleucine and tryptophan have been found to be low in anorexia patients. Supplementing valine, and isoleucine help to build muscle

In broad terms giving a free-form amino acid supplement is probably the best strategy for building muscle - plus the inclusion of zinc, B6 and digestive enzymes. The ideal diet should include easily assimilable foods containing good quality protein such as quinoa, fish, soya and spirulina or blue-green algae. Other good foods are ground seeds, lentils, beans, plus fruits and vegetables.

Bulimia

Bulimia is binge eating followed by self-induced vomiting and is probably a more common condition nowadays. Some anorexics are bulimic. Some bulimics are not anorexic. It is still a food/weight compulsive/obsessive disorder. It is classified as follows:

A Recurrent episodes of binge eating (rapid consumption of large amounts of food in a discrete period of time)
B A feeling of lack of control over eating behaviour during the eating binges.
C The person regularly engages in self-induced vomiting, use of laxatives, diuretics, strict dieting, fasting, or exercise in order to prevent weight gain.
D A minimum average of two binge eating sessions a week.
E Persistent overconcern with body shape and weight.

Zinc is again important to consider. Although amino acid depletion, unless anorexic, would appear less likely, full spectrum amino acid supplementation does seem to help. Food allergies/addictions, hypoglycemia, and candidiasis are biochemical imbalances than may well contribute to this pattern of behaviour. Nutritional strategies are most effective if given alongside counselling as psychological issues are almost always playing a part.

Summary of Research Linking Zinc & Anorexia

1973, Hambidge and Silverman, concluded that, **"whenever there is appetite loss in children zinc deficiency should be suspected"** Arch. Dis. Child, 48, 567

1979, Bakan, concluded that **"the symptoms of anorexia and zinc deficiency are similar in a number of respects... It is proposed that clinical trials be undertaken to test its effectiveness in treatment"** Med. Hyp. 5,7

1980, Horrobin et al concluded **"There is substantial evidence to suggest that anorexia nervosa is due to a combined deficiency of zinc and EFA's."** Med. Hyp. 6, p.277-296

1980, Casper & Prasad, concluded **"10/13 patients with anorexia and 8/14 patients with bulimia were zinc deficient on admission. Patients with anorexia nervosa undergoing vigourous refeeding should receive zinc supplementation because of the high risk of developing zinc deficiency during this period of anabolism and presumably increased zinc demands."**

1984, Flanagan, concluded **"An early effect of zinc deficiency in rats is loss of appetite.... rats tube fed a zinc deficient diet thrived for 6-7 days then became seriously ill"** J.Nutr. 114, p.493-502

1984, Bryce-Smith & Simpson report **"Within 2 months (of zinc supplementation of 45mg p.d) her weight returned (from 31.5kg) to 44.5kg, she was cheerful again, and the taste test was strongly positive."** Lancet, August 11, p.350-351

1984, Akar report **"small intestinal mucosal abnormality is completely restored to normal after oral zinc therapy. In cases of anorexia nervosa it is worth looking for small-intestinal mucosal changes."** Lancet, October 13, p.874

1985, Karsaskis et al, concluded **"We propose that during zinc deficiency, a reduction in the receptor affinity for noradrenalin may occur and might represent a primary deficit responsible for reduced food intake in this condition."** Biol. Tace. Elem. Res. 9, p.25

1985, Dinsmore et al, concluded **"our data provide further evidence of a disturbance in zinc metabolism (absorption?) in anorexia nervosa"** Lancet, May 4, p.1040-1

1986, Safai-Kutti, reported **"Our initial patient is currently maintained on zinc supplementation (45mg p.d.). She is doing very** well: her weight as well as her menstruations are normalised." Am.J.Clin.Nut. 44, p.581-582

1986, Jonas & Gold reported **"An accumulating body of evidence suggests a link between substance abuse and eating disorders"** Lancet, Feb 15, p.390

1986, Ward concluded **"The urinary element content of a 21-year-old female suffering from anorexia nervosa exhibits highly significant decreases in Ca, Co, Cr, Cu, Fe and Zn when compared to an age matched female control. Zinc, and possibly calcium imbalance is shown to be associated with anorexia nervosa."** J.Micronut.Anal. 2, p.211-231

1987, Katz et al, concluded from a double-blind randomised trial of 15 anorexic patients **"Zinc supplementation was followed by a decrease in depression and anxiety..Our data suggest that individuals with anorexia nervosa may be at risk for zinc deficiency and may respond favourably after zinc supplementation."** J.Adol.Health Care, 8, p.400-406

1989, Humphries et al, concluded **"40% of patients with bulimia (n=62) and 54% of those with anorexia nervosa(n=24) had biochemical evidence of zinc deficiency."** J.Clin.Psych. 50,12,p.456-459

1990, Ward concluded **"A statistically significant difference (p<0.001) in zinc content (anorexic/15 < control/15) was seen in whole blood, blood serum, plasma, urine and washed scalp hair."** J.Nut.Med. 1,p.171-178

1990, Safai-Kutti reported, in an open study **"During a follow-up period of 8-56 months 17 out of 20 patients increased their body weight by more than 15%. The maximal weight gain was 57% after 24 months of zinc therapy. The most rapid weight gain was 24% over 3 months. None had weight loss after the administration of zinc therapy. None of our patients developed bulimia."** Acta Psychiatr Scand Suppl 361, p14-17

1994, Birmingham et al, carried out a double-blind controlled trial giving 100mg of zinc gluconate and concluded **"The rate of increase in BMI of the zinc supplemented group was twice that of the placebo group and this difference was statistically significant (p=0.03)."** Int.J.Eat.Disord. 15 (3), p251-55.

25

PREVENTING PREMATURE SENILITY

Senility is described as a 'mental disease in which brain cells cease to function properly, resulting in a deficit in memory and mental capability'. The size of the problem is on the increase. One in four people over 75, and one in seven over 65, are classified as senile. In fact, a third of all hospital beds are filled with geriatrics, a large proportion of them institutionalised because of senility. The cost to the taxpayer runs into billions.

What is Senility?

To understand senility we must examine the nature of memory. In a lifetime, more than 15 trillion specific memories are coded in our brain. Although much of what we perceive is forgotten, selected glimpses remain permanently etched, waiting for recall. So memory can be divided into short-term (lasting a few seconds or minutes) or long-term.

Memory Theories

Two current theories exist. One involves coding through lipoproteins, fat containing proteins in the brain. In fact, every cell in our brain contains special kinds of fat, which can be synthesised only from the essential fatty acids linoleic and linolenic acid. Synthesis of these is made even easier by the intake of essential fatty acids found in fatty fish, high in EPA, or in seeds and their oil, such as evening primrose oil, high in GLA.

The other theory is based on coding through RNA, the messenger molecule in charge of building new cells.Since most of the brain cells are replaced within twenty-four hours, the clue to memory must be transmittable. Foods high in RNA, like fish, have been shown to boost mental activity and memory in animals.

Research at the Princeton Bio Center has shown a link between senile dementia and the polyamine spermine - which the brain badly needs to make more RNA [1]. The minerals zinc and, most importantly, manganese help to bring low spermine levels back to normal.

The Aluminium Connection

One common finding is that premature senile dementia, known as Alzheimer's disease, is an entanglement of nerve fibres. When these nerve clusters are found in the frontal and temporal regions of the brain they are frequently loaded with aluminium [2]. One possibility is that the involuntary consumption of aluminium contributes to deteriorating memory and mental performance. We get aluminium from cooking utensils and food packaging, including aluminium foil. People with indigestion risk an extra dose from many types of antacids.

Another hypothesis is that the nerve cells are simply not getting enough blood. The brain uses a fifth of your blood supply. Most people by the age of 50 have a degree of arteriosclerosis and atherosclerosis - hardening and 'furring up' of the arteries. In severe cases this leads to a stroke, where the whole blood supply to a portion of the brain is cut off. The result is death of partial paralysis. When cells are starved of oxygen they switch to a more primitive mode of operation called anaerobic respiration. The cells begin to divide and spread - unless they are nerve cells, that is, because nerve cells can't regenerate. So what happens to them? They just stop working. The result is senility.

Oxygen boosters

To keep cells running on oxygen requires much more than a good blood supply. Vitamins are also involved in the process of oxygen and energy metabolism. The most important are vitamins B1 and B3 and the antioxidant vitamins A, C, E and the mineral selenium.

Vitamin B1 deficiency has long been known to result in brain damage. One of the most dangerous problems of excessive alcohol consumption is induced B1 deficiency. The condition is called Wernicke-Korsakof syndrome. The symptoms include anxiety and depression, obsessive thinking, confusion, defective memory (especially from recent events) and time distortion - not so different from senility.

Vitamin B3, also known as niacin, is crucial for oxygen utilisation. It is incorporated into the coenzyme NAD (nicotinamide adenosine dinucleotide), and many reactions involving oxygen need NAD. Without it, pellagra and senility can develop.

Memory Boosters

Other memory boosters include B vitamins, especially choline. This nutrient probably works by boosting the levels of acetylcholine, an important nerve transmitter substance. In studies at the Palo Alto Hospital in California, drugs which boost acetylcholine induced 'supermemories'. Choline on its own is effective in improving short-term and long-term memory, but the doses have to be high (10 grams a day) and the effects are not very long lasting. Pantothenic acid, B5, is also important in acetylcholine synthesis. Deanol, which is a salt of DMAE, is a more effective choline derivative which easily passes all membrane barriers. The dose is only 100mg per day, rather than 10g as with choline. DMAE, a nutrient found in fish, can also be taken at a level of 500mg a day.

Another potential memory booster is an amino acid called pyroglutamate which is found in fruit and vegetables. The discovery that the brain and cerebrospinal fluid contains large amounts of pyroglutamate led to it's investigation as an essential brain nutrient. Doctors prescribe nootropics to millions of people every year for memory deficit problems. Their basic effect is to improve learning, memory consolidation, and memory retrieval with no toxicity or side-effects. One study, published in 1988 by Dr Pilch and colleagues, suggests that nootropics may increase the number of acetylcholine receptors in the brain [3]. Older mice were given piracetam, a pyroglutamate derivative, for two weeks. The researchers found that these older mice had 30-40% higher density of receptors than before. This suggests that pyroglutamate-like molecules may also have a regenerative effect on the nervous system.

The effects of enhancing mental performance through supplementation of 'smart nutrients' such as phosphatidyl choline, pantothenic acid, DMAE and pyroglutamate are likely to be far greater when taken in combination than individually. In one study in 1981, a team of researchers led by Raymond Bartus gave choline and piracetam, a pyroglutamate derivative, to aged lab rats noted for age-related memory decline [4]. They found that "rats given the piracetam/choline combination exhibited (memory) retention scores several times better than those with piracetam alone." They found that half the dose was needed when piracetam and choline were combined. A good strategy for treating memory deficit should include these nutrients plus all-round optimum nutrition.

Optimum Nutrition

But don't the elderly get enough of these vital vitamins? Sadly the answer is unequivocal 'no'. And anyway enough is not always enough. Dr. Abram Hoffer has shown that when cells have been starved of these nutrients they may become vitamin dependent, requiring many hundred times the normal daily requirements.

One study in the States in 1975 failed to find a single geriatric patient with a normal nutritional profile! [5] The most common deficiencies were C, E, A and B3. Other studies have found the elderly to be frequently deficient in folic acid, zinc, iron and of course calcium. To prevent the risk of heart and artery disease many researchers have recommended low-fat diets, cutting down on dairy produce and meat. This often leads to even worse iron, zinc and calcium status, unless proper dietary guidance and supplementation is given. Many elderly people have impaired sense of taste, leading to over-salting of food.

Senility and Alzheimer's disease may prove to be the consequence of decades of sub-optimal nutrition. With optimum nutrition I believe senility and memory deterioration will become a thing of the past. As Leonard Larson, president of the American Medical Association in 1960, said, 'There is no diseases of the aged, but simply diseases among the aged'.

26

SOLVING SLEEPING PROBLEMS

One of the the great mysteries is why we need sleep at all. Without it, even for a night, the body shows clear signs of stress. Zinc and magnesium levels drop, vitamin C is used up at an alarming rate and when there is a chance to catch up on lost sleep, providing we are healthy, we very quickly enter an intensive kind of sleep called REM (Rapid Eye Movement) sleep. REM sleep normally occurs 90 minutes after sleep onset, but if we are sleep deprived it may occur within 30 minutes.

Dreaming occurs during REM sleep and most of us have four or more REM periods per night even though many people have difficulty remembering the dreams which occur in them. As well as providing a physical rest, sleep may provide a chance to make a 'back up tape' of the day's events for our large computer, the brain. While westerners pay little heed to dreams, one African tribe believe 'real life' is lived in dreams and daytime is the illusion. The Bolivian philosopher Oscar Ichazo, described dream reality like the stars at night: that dream thoughts are always happening, but the brightness of the sun, daytime consciousness, blots them out. Many scientists believe that dreaming is normal and that nutritional deficiency is one reason why poor or no dream recall can occur. In a survey at ION we found that more 40% of people had no or very infrequent dream recall. When researching the signs and symptoms of vitamin B6 and zinc deficiency we found that an alarming proportion of deficient people couldn't recall their dreams. After supplementation with B6 and zinc, often in doses as high as 1,000mg of B6 and 100mg of zinc, dream recall would return. If they took too much B6 and zinc dreams became too vivid and the person would wake up in the night. Vitamin B6 and zinc also affected the quality of dreams.

So if you don't think you dream it's worth supplementing B6 and zinc, gradually increasing the dose up to 500mg B6 and 50mg of zinc. (It is best not to take more without the advice of a nutritionist).

But far more serious than lack of dream recall is insomnia. Most people at some time in their lives, have experienced the frustration, restlessness and exhaustion that occurs when they either can't get enough sleep or wake up too early and can't get back to sleep. This is perhaps understandable at times of great stress or worry, but can also be effected by what you eat.

The process of falling to sleep happens as a result of levels of the brain nerve-transmitter serotonin rising and levels of circulating adrenalin decreasing. Serotonin is partly made from the protein constituent tryptophan. This is converted in the presence of B6 first into B3 and then into serotonin. Adequate amounts of B6 and tryptophan are needed to get sleepy. Some foods, like turkey for example, are particularly high in tryptophan, which may help to explain why everybody falls asleep after Christmas dinner. Supplementing one to four tablets of l-tryptophan 500mg helps to induce sleep, but this must be taken an hour before the intended 'departure time' without food.

For some it is not so much the level of serotonin that is a problem but that they are over-stimulated and perhaps over-anxious. These are the light sleepers and early wakers. Vitamin B6 and the minerals calcium and magnesium are nature's tranquillisers. They calm down nerve activity and can help to give a better night's sleep (as well as preventing night cramps). Levels of at least 100mg of B6, 600mg calcium and 400mg magnesium are usually needed to produce a result. It is best to use highly bioavailable forms of these minerals such as citrates or amino acid chelates. While foods like sesame seeds, almonds and green leafy vegetables are excellent sources of calcium and magnesium, just changing the diet is rarely effective in dealing with insomnia in the short term. Dolomite tablets contain the right balance of calcium and magnesium.

Stimulants like tea, coffee, sugar, cola, chocolate and cigarettes can knock out the calming effects of these tranquillising nutrients so must be strictly avoided, especially in the evening. Instead drink herb teas, many of which have their own calming effect. Milk drinks may also be calming, but not if they contain chocolate. Interestingly, the coffee berry

---

Sleep - Are You Getting Enough?

Most people spend a third of their life asleep. If you're not getting your share here's how to fall asleep and stay asleep:

- Supplement B6 100mg + Zinc 10mg (up to 50mg if no dream recall)
- Supplement 600mg of calcium and 400mg of magnesium in the evening
- Avoid all stimulants after 4pm
- Take 1 to 2 x l-tryptophan 1,000mg (if still necessary)*
- Eat calcium and magnesium rich foods

---

that surrounds the coffee bean is a relaxant while the bean is a stimulant, which illustrates how natural foods are often balanced and refined foods are not.

*At the time of writing the essential amino acid tryptophan is, however, not available for free sale, having been banned in 1989 due a contaminant introduced through its production by genetic engineering. Tryptophan, which has been used for years as a safe, non-addictive alternative to sleeping pills, is currently only available on prescription as Optimax produced by the pharmaceutical company, Merck.

But, you might think, if it is now classified as safe, why has the ban on tryptophan sale as a nutritional supplement not been lifted? This question has yet to be satisfactorily answered by UK and US health officials.

27

FITS, CONVULSIONS AND EPILEPSY

While teaching classes in Oxford, Francis had a bad car accident. This left him with severe headaches, poor memory and concentration, severe depression but most of all, epilepsy. So bad was his epilepsy that he complained of 'epileptic storms' sometimes daily. During the night he would often have five or six fits, despite being on anti-epilepsy drugs. His memory had so deteriorated he could no longer teach, and being epileptic he found it hard to get work. Naturally he became depressed.

After years under medical supervision he decided to try some alternatives and was referred to me. He promised to avoid tea, coffee and sugar and we discussed how to eat a balanced diet, with plenty of fruit, vegetables and wholegrains - the 'optimum' diet.

I wanted to give him every chance to change and included high levels of supplements giving him B3, B5 and B6, choline, calcium, zinc, magnesium and manganese as well as other nutrients. Magnesium and manganese have both been shown to help epilepsy, while B5 and choline have a specific effect on memory.

When he came back after one month, he had made tremendous changes to his diet and had reaped the rewards of his efforts. "I am amazed at how well I feel" he commented and told me he hadn't had a single muscle tremor or panic attack. Three months later he had still only had one epileptic 'storm'. His brain is working better, his depression gone and he can sleep straight through the night, without any fits or muscle tremors. (Case supplied by Christopher Scarfe)

Differences in the nutritional status of those with fits or epilepsy, and those without has been demonstrated by many researchers. The two key minerals that have frequently been shown to be deficient are manganese and magnesium.

The Mineral Connection

Manganese is essential for proper brain function and, to date, four studies have shown a correlation between low levels and the presence of epilepsy [1,2,3,4]. Supplementing manganese helped to reduce fits. In one study published in the Journal of the American Medical Association one child had half the normal blood manganese levels[x]. He didn't respond to any medication, but, on supplementing manganese, he had fewer seizures and improved speech and learning. We have frequently found that patients with convulsions or fits are manganese deficient and have no or fewer fits once supplementation is started.

Manganese was first used by Dr Kunin to treat drug induced muscular spasms, called tardive dyskinesia. He treated fifteen such cases, seven of which were completely relieved of symptoms and only one showed no improvement.

Magnesium is also vital for proper nerve and brain function. Once again, a number of researchers have found low levels in patients with epilepsy and reported less fits on supplementation. Magnesium injections may be able to instantly suppress convulsions.

Other key nutrients linked with fits and convulsion are vitamin B6 and zinc. Anticonvulsants can rob the body of zinc either by reducing absorption, by binding to the zinc or by causing diarrheoa. In any case extra zinc is recommended.

It's best to have a mineral deficiency screening test, such as a hair mineral analysis, to find out if there are any deficiencies. Once these are corrected fits often stop.

As anticonvulsant drugs often deplete folic acid, some researchers have also supplemented folic acid [5,6]. The results have not always been good. In some cases folic acid supplementation has resulted in more fits. So care needs to be exercised with folic acid supplementation, preferably only after blood tests have confirmed deficiency.

There have also been reports of improvement once food allergens are removed [7,8,9], so it's well worth investigating this possibility.

28

MOOD SWINGS AND MANIC DEPRESSION

Monica had a long history of mental illness. She had spent most of her life on drugs and had even been given a lobotomy. While these treatments sedated her she continually suffered from depression and occasional 'highs'. At the age of 70 she consulted a nutrition counsellor. At this point she was on two drugs - Depixol injections and Flupenthixol. She had side-effects from the drugs, as well as high blood pressure. Her nutrition counsellor identified nutritional deficiencies. As soon as these were corrected the depression lifted. She was able to stop one drug and halve the dose of Depixol. With this she continued to improve and had reduced drug side-effects. Her blood pressure stabilised so that she stopped medication for this too. She no longer has 'highs', nor depression and, for the first time in as long as she remembers, feels normal.

Without a doubt, some families have relatives who seasonally get the blues or fly so high in their moods that they literally give away their home. If the high mood is controllable they work day and night and make enough money to afford to spend their depressed moods in a luxury hotel. There the doctor in residence eventually gets to know the whole family and gives encouragement and appropriate treatment. As time passes, the elevated productive mood returns and the victim of manic-depression goes back to work. Compared to other mental disorders the manic-depressive mood change is rather noble since we remember the mood changes in the kings of Shakespeare's tragedies. This illness occurs most often in colour-blind males who also have O-type blood. Like haemophilia, the disorder is linked to the X chromosome, so many women are carriers of the disorder. Manic-depression was presumably not adequately named so psychiatrists introduced the useless term 'bipolar disorder' for the manic-depressive patient. Those who only get depressed periodically are now labelled 'mono-polar disorder' patients.

Understanding Cyclical Mood Changes

The most common mood change is that which occurs daily. Some people learn early in life that they are 'morning larks', while others do their best work at night and are 'night owls'. These pairs make unlikely room-mates and equally mismatched mates in marriage. The morning cup of caffeine (tea or coffee) will chase the morning blues and overdosage may produce jitters and manic behaviour. If mood changes are not owing to drug intake (caffeine, alcohol, cocaine), then the possibility of food allergy or hypoglycemia should be carefully investigated. Dr. Walter Alvarez, in the 1920's first found that his blue Mondays occurred because his family were rich enough to have chicken every Sunday. When he avoided chicken on Sunday, his Mondays were once again productive. Thus daily or even day-to-day mood changes are almost always due to food allergies or hypoglycemia. Some patients are affected by the sun and feel better at night, when the sun is behind the earth. They get jobs as cooks in all-night restaurants or sort the cheques for the banks at night.

Weekly mood changes can be correlated with the work pattern of a seven-day week. Many migraine patients have depression and headaches at the weekend. This is called relaxation headache and the migraine sufferer may therefore never get to rest and evolves into the 'Type A' personality that seldom relaxes - the workaholic. Excessive stress may dissipate all zinc and B6 so that the person becomes pyroluric and has excessive mood swings. Most of the patients who come to the Princeton Bio Center with a diagnosis of manic-depression and have weekly swings in mood are merely pyroluric. They are easily treated with adequate zinc and B6. Monthly mood changes can be correlated with hormonal changes in the female and moon phases in both sexes. Much has been written about premenstrual tension, but it is not generally known that the tension occurs when blood copper is highest and the blood zinc is lowest. Copper is a stimulant to the brain, while zinc has an anti-anxiety effect. This metal imbalance reverses at the onset of menstruation, often coinciding with relief of tension and other symptoms. Another mineral of potential interest is vanadium. This trace element affects levels of monoamines in the brain and, according to one study by Professor Derek Bryce-Smith and Dr Naylor, manic patients have raised levels which fall on recovery [1]. They also found that giving agents which lower vanadium concentration, such as ascorbic acid, helped those with mania and depression [2]. However, not all studies have reported the same benefits.

Much has been written about the lunar (moon) effect from which we originally got the word 'lunacy' and 'lunatic'. One only has to consider the powerful effect the moon has in creating tides to realise that each one of us (we are, after all, 66% water) is also affected by the moon. Seasonal, as well as monthly changes in mood are well known. Peptic ulcers tend to be activated in the spring and autumn, inhalant allergy is more common in the spring with trees and grass pollen, and in the autumn with weed pollens. The allergic patients learn early in life about seasonal tormentors. Springtime is a period of increased energy and growth in the northern hemisphere so appropriate stresses and bodily changes are to be expected.

Another possible factor is light. Some people suffer depression only in the winter and are diagnosed with S.A.D.-seasonally affected depression. Since light has a powerful effect on brain hormone balance experimental treatments elongating the daylight hours by using light boxes do produce beneficial results in some SAD patients [3].

Some patients are depressed during their entire life. These patients are either deficient in thyroid function or high in histamine, or both. A trial of thyroid usually allows them to get over their daily depression. A blood analysis for the histamine level or a basophil count will establish the presence of a high level of blood histamine. The avoidance of folic acid and the use of daily methionine (an amino acid) will dispel their daily depression.

Lithium - an Effective Treatment for Mania

Lithium therapy for over-excited patients was discovered in 1949 by Dr. John Cape of Australia, but medical acceptance has been slow. For instance, lithium therapy for the treatment only of the manic stage of manic-depressive disorders was started in 1970. Because of the excellent studies of a Danish investigator, Dr. Schau, lithium therapy has been available since 1960 in Denmark and other countries 4. Numerous publications have appeared indicating that lithium therapy is also useful in the treatment of chronic depression, alcoholism, premenstrual depression and hyperthyroidism.

Dr. Manfred Anke, then of the Karl Marx Veterinary School of Leipzig, Germany, found that lithium is an essential element needed by the goat and the miniature pig. (This discovery, if extended to man, may mean that psychiatrists who prescribe lithium are, unwittingly, meganutrient therapists!) Lithium-deficient animals lie dormant with no muscle tone. This finding needs to be confirmed since we have many patients who have only a trace of lithium in their hair and may therefore benefit from supplementing lithium.

We have used lithium in schizophrenic and other patients for a period of fifteen years. We know that lithium has no effect on hallucinations, but lithium does allow the non-hallucinatory patients to reduce his effective anti-psychotic drug dose. The side effects of large doses of Prolixin are therefore diminished. The patient is also better able to tolerate hallucinations while on lithium therapy.

Lithium is specific, according to Dr. Levy 5. "The patient receiving lithium treatment is alert without lethargy or sedation. It seems clear that lithium is the ideal therapeutic agent for acute and chronic mania. It is also very effective for the hypomanic states whose frequent recurrence leads to deterioration of the patient's social situation. In this type of patient, lithium is superior to other drugs which produce only brief symptomatic improvement and a large amount of sedation."

Low doses of Lithium can Relieve Depression

What has caused even more interest in lithium is that it appears to be active as a prophylactic agent against recurrent psychotic depression. Studies have shown that lithium given on an ongoing basis in smaller does to patients with recurrent depression is able to substantially diminish the depressive attacks. The fact holds true whether the patient has shown only depression in the past or has had alternating phases of mania and depression. If used on a regular basis, lithium requires a dosage with a few side-effects and causes no restriction of normal emotional expression.

Some professionals motivated by inexperience (and their desire to fill hospital beds) tell the patient that 'Lithium therapy can only be started in a hospital where daily lithium levels will be run.' This is untrue! We, and others, have found that patients between the ages of 12 and 50 years can be started on two 300mg tablets of lithium carbonate per day. (The mean lithium level produced by this low dose therapy is 0.4 meg/1. The recommended therapeutic level for mania is 0.5-1.5 meg/1. Therefore, we are well below the level that might produce any untoward reaction). We sometimes suggest that the patient, if unimproved, start lithium therapy (two tablets per day) two weeks before the next scheduled visit. We then do a blood serum lithium level.

What are the Side-Effects?

The side-effects depend on the dosage used. One or two tablets or capsules per day (American tablets contain 300mg lithium carbonate; European contain 400mg) may produce a fine tremor of the hands, slight tiredness and sleepiness. Three to four tablets or capsules a day can bring on nausea, diarrhoea, increased thirst and urination, and low thyroid function.

Lithium is compatible with all of the tranquillisers, vitamins, nutrients and antibiotics when the dose is small. Some reports indicate that haloperidol (Haldol) and lithium provide a sometimes lethal combination when given in large doses. This is true of any major tranquilliser with large doses of lithium. Lithium should not be recommended for patients on digitalis or diuretic pills.

Advantages of Lithium Therapy

Because lithium is excreted slowly from the body, this means that a therapeutic level is maintained longer and also allows simple blood tests for lithium to determine whether the patient is sticking to the treatment. At high levels lithium causes nausea and vomiting, which means that patients are unlikely to overdose. In conjunction with good nutrition, lithium is a viable alternative to the more dangerous drugs commonly used for manic-depressed and chronically depressed people.

Part 5

THE ACTION PLAN FOR MENTAL HEALTH

Procrastination, she said, was the source of all my sorrow. I don't know what the word means. I'll look it up tomorrow.

29

GETTING OFF DRUGS

Since the 1950s the treatment of mental illness with drugs has become the major therapeutic tool of psychiatrists the world over. The first anti-psychotic drug, reserpine, was introduced into psychiatric practice in 1952, shortly followed by chlorpromazine (Thorazine) in 1954. The perfecting of this type of anti-psychotic drug was achieved in the 1960s with the introduction of fluphenazine (Prolixin) and haloperidol (Haldol). Most other anti-psychotic drugs introduced since 1970 have been 'me too' drugs which have little advantage over these two standard and now cheaper drugs. For patients who will not co-operate on the taking of medication by mouth, the oil-soluble decanoate salts are available for intramuscular injection. These weekly injections - for example, of Depixol - do not give as smooth a result as the daily use of the drug by mouth. Most patients can have the daily dose they need given by mouth at bedtime with dephenhydramine (Benadryl). If an antidote to any muscle shakes (side action) is needed, Cogentin, Artane or Kemadrin can be given in a small dose each morning.

Drugs such as the major tranquillisers should only be considered as temporary crutches which can be used until the biochemical imbalances are slowly corrected by nutrient therapy. Anti-psychotic drugs, if continued at high doses for many months, may produce tardive dyskinesia - a delayed impairment of voluntary motion causing incomplete or partial movement. The risk of getting tardive dyskinesia is 75 per cent, after long-term use, according to Dr William Glazer, an expert on tardive dyskinesia. Manganese taken daily in doses of 50mg is helpful, as is the daily use of Deanol which builds up acetylcholine, the normal working hormone in muscle contraction.

Another problem is multiple drug interactions. Many psychiatric patients take, simultaneously, daily doses of one or more anti-psychotics, anti-depressants, a minor tranquilliser and a hypnotic to make them sleep at night. In addition, because of certain side effects of these drugs, which resemble the symptoms off Parkinson's Disease, most patients are given an atropine-like drug (anti-Parkinson agent) such as Cogentin or Kemadrin. These make the reading of the printed page even more difficult. Then there are drugs for co-existing illnesses prescribed by other doctors and self-medication with over-the-counter drugs, all of which the patient could conceivably take simultaneously. All this adds up to a potentially dangerous constellation of pharmacological interaction and personal neglect of the patient which might prolong suffering and delay rehabilitation.

Studies have indicated that only a few patients on anti-psychotic drugs require an anti-Parkinson drug for a prolonged period. And while anti-psychotic drugs can have beneficial short-term effects, the lethargic, asocial, odd behaviour of some patients, which is usually attributed to illness, may well be the result of medication.

When San Francisco Examiner columnist, Bill Mandel, tried 50mg of Thorazine he reported, "Simply put, it made me stupid. Because Thorazine and related drugs are called 'liquid lobotomy' in the mental health business, I'd expected a great grey cloud to descend over my faculties. There was no grey cloud, just small, unsettling patches of fog. My mental gears slipped. I had no intellectual traction. It was difficult to remember simple words." Most patients are prescribed 2 to 16 times the amount taken by Mandel. In these patients, when dosages are reduced or drugs discontinued, a favourable transformation occurs as the patients become more social and much of the odd behaviour disappears.

Often the wrong drugs are recommended. There are many reasons why this could occur, such as understaffing in hospitals, lack of interaction between patient and doctor, discrepancies between scientific understanding and clinical use, and the effects of drug advertising, which may not serve the best interests of responsible medical practice. Whatever the cause, it is important that the patient knows there are viable alternatives to choose from. Adequate diagnosis combined with an optimum diet plus specific nutrients are the first steps towards a more effective and tolerable treatment. If needed, a drug such as haloperidol or fluphenazine may be substituted for chlorpromazine. These produce fewer side-effects, but should only be used as 'holding drugs' until the nutrients begin to take effect. A 'pharmacological lobotomy' is not necessary, nor is the frustrating disruption of patients' imaginative resources.

The Danger of Long-term Drug Abuse

Prolonged use of haloperidol or fluphenazine (without extra nutrients) can, and usually does result in tardive dyskinesia. The nutrients which will help prevent this chronic illness are manganese with choline or Deanol which, as we have already seen, is a precursor for acetylcholine, an important neurotransmitter. Once the disorder has appeared, the use of choline, Deanol and manganese may take weeks or months to correct the abnormal movements caused by tardive dyskinesia. Vitamin E may also help, at a level of 800ius per day. [1]

The 'neuroleptic malignant syndrome' is yet another sometimes lethal side-effect of anti-schizophrenic medication. More than twenty publications have depicted the sad effects of prolonged use of the anti-schizophrenic drugs. Patients may get elevated temperature, sweating, rapid pulse, panting, soiling, rigidity, stupor and coma. If the drug is not withdrawn, death can occur within twenty-four hours.

Drugs can have Serious Side-effects

A problem which has been overlooked in the treatment of mental disorders until recently is the discomfort to the patient resulting from the side-effects of some psychotherapeutic drugs. Drugs such as the now antiquated chlorpromazine, (Thorazine or Largactil) can have some annoying and sometimes serious side-effects. Patients taking these drugs may find themselves unable to steady their hands; their facial muscles may twitch involuntarily; they may try to read but find their vision is too blurred to decipher the printed lines. The eyes may turn up and refuse to come down. The patients may be restless and pace the floor until they have blistered feet. A severe skin reaction may follow even a brief exposure to the sun so that patients on the drug are compelled to spend much of their time indoors. After long-term drug therapy a patient may look in the mirror one morning to discover that his face has acquired a purplish-grey hue, a very slowly reversible condition. This pigment is also in the heart muscle and may cause sudden death, as several studies have shown. An intelligent young man or woman, particularly the artistic or intellectual type, may make the frustrating discovery that their much valued imaginative facilities are no longer available. Is is ethical, twenty five years after the introduction of chlorpromazine, to increase the agony of the suffering schizophrenic by giving him this drug when safer drugs are available? With newer and better drugs, and improved methods of treating the schizophrenias through nutrition, any informed medical doctor should know that chlorpromazine is antiquated. Yet some psychiatric consultants will prescribe it only because it is the oldest tranquilliser.

Anti-depressant drugs are also not without risk. Trycyclic antidepressants such as Amitriptyline, Anafranil and Prothiadin, have over 20 side-effects listed in the doctor's drug guide, the British National Formulary, including dry mouth, blurred vision, nausea, confusion, cardiovascular problems, sweating, tremors and behavioural disturbance [2]. Mono-amine oxidase inhibitors, called MAOI's, such as Nardil and Parstelin, have even worse side-effects and can be very difficult to come off as they are highly addictive. Deaths have occurred from pateints taking MAOI's and not avoiding alcohol or certain foods, like cheese and yeast, both found hidden in many convenience foods. The new class of anti-depressants that work by inhibiting the uptake of serotonin are touted as having less side-effects for most, but can create profound problems. Prozac, the market leader, with sales in excess of $1 billion a year, has 45 side-effects listed in the British national Formulary [3]. Since its release in 1987 there have been 160 lawsuits brought against its manufacture over alleged violent or suicidal reactions [4]. According to psychiatrist, David Richman, between 10 and 25 per cent of people experienced each of the following: nausea, nervousness, insomnia, headache, tremors, anxiety, drowsiness, dry mouth, excessive sweating and diarrhoea. Somewhat better tolerated is Lustral, or sertraline. Anti-depressant sshould be used only as a last resort, and even then, for a short period of time.

According to Dr Abram Hoffer, a psychiatrist with 40 years of experience in treating mental illness, tranquillisers never cure mental illness because tranquillisers replace one psychosis with another [5]. No normal person can function under the influence of tranquillisers. Yet even today, one unfortunate consequence of understaffing of public mental hospitals is that excessive doses of chlorpromazine are routinely prescribed to keep the patient quiet. Medical supervision is minimal and treatment is not monitored properly. Chlorpromazine is also cheaper, which appeals to the economy-minded purchasing agent of the hospital. Tranquillisers should only be used as a last resort, and even then, phased out as the patient improves on the right nutrients.

30

FINDING HELP AND STAYING OUT OF HOSPITAL

Help is widely available all over Britain. Many nutrition counsellors (sometimes called nutrition consultants, dietary therapists, dieticians or nutritionists) are available for guidance. Most nutrition counsellors are in private practice and charge around £30 for an initial consultation which usually lasts for an hour. Some medical practices can refer you to a dietician on the NHS, however few are trained in the orthomolecular approach.

A nationwide Directory of Nutrition Counsellors is available for £2 (inc. p&p) from The Institute for Optimum Nutrition, Blades Court, Deodar Road, London SW15 2NU Tel: 0181 877 9993 Fax: 0181 877 9980.

Some nutrition counsellors are more experienced than others in the field of mental health and nutrition so it is best to ask them if they can help you. If not, they can refer you to another nutrition counsellor who specialises in mental health problems. In case of difficulty please contact the Institute for Optimum Nutrition which runs post-graduate courses in mental health and nutrition and can put you in touch with your nearest suitably qualified nutrition counsellor.

Half-Way Houses better than Hospitals

Hospitals seldom follow the directions of orthomolecular practitioners. Thus intake of the essential nutrients is frequently stopped on entering psychiatric hospitals. Without the essential nutrients, which are known to be needed, the patient rapidly relapses and hospitalisation is prolonged. What's more, hospital diets usually include wheat, sugar, dairy produce and large amounts of tea and coffee, none of which are going to help recovery.

Suitable alternatives to hospitalisation must be provided. The alternatives may range from halfway houses to treatment in the home under care of an operative nurse trained in the orthomolecular approach. Parents or relatives can also give orthomolecular care. The orthomolecular practitioner can thus continue to provide the medical care. This situation is similar to childbirth under the care of a wise midwife with the trained doctor available on call. The overall result is better and the patient will make continuous progress toward recovery from the cerebral allergy or illness.

The halfway house takes years of effort to establish. The usual population of patients at any one time will vary from six to twenty patients. Plans must be made for proper food, nonallergic housing, daily care and exercise and dismissal of patients. The houses will not make a profit so it should be organised as a not-for-profit unit and should receive help from government bodies or annual donations from benefactors. The insurance companies should pay for this care as they do for hospital care. Some voluntary help can be used to ease the great financial burden.

Rosalind la Roche, who now runs Earth House in New Jersey, USA, was the first trained operative in the field of orthomolecular medicine. She heard, at a reception of a recluse schizophrenic brother of a famous psychiatrist. She suggested that with her orthomolecular nutritional knowledge she could socially rehabilitate the recluse brother. She travelled halfway across America with packets of nutrients and within two months she had the recluse exercising daily and working at the family factory. He is now totally rehabilitated and is a member of the board of directors of Earth House. Such activity needs courage, strength, self-assurance and adequate training on the part of the orthomolecular operative. This training can be had at some of the orthomolecular centres around the world. Patients who cannot be left alone or patients who have withdrawn from society are the prime targets for therapy supervised by operatives.

As an alternative to the halfway house, a trained psychiatric nurse may agree to take a patient into her home for continued therapy. We have found this type of orthomolecular therapy to be highly successful and perhaps the least expensive of any arrangement. The new family milieu is particularly conducive to rehabilitation. It is obvious that any of these options are better than the psychiatric hospital or the rented bare apartment which is frequently suggested to get the patient away from the family. Premature isolation of the patient will result in malnutrition and the loneliness may lead to suicide.

31

DIET AND SUPPLEMENTS FOR MENTAL HEALTH

The nutritional approach to mental illness is more 'labour intensive' than taking prescribed drugs. It requires gradual changes to lifelong habits. For this reason proper professional support from a nutrition counsellor, backed up by support and encouragement from family and friends, is essential. Nutrition counsellors are trained to identify if a person has allergies, glucose intolerance, nutrient deficiencies or anti-nutrient excesses. A lot of time can be saved by getting an accurate diagnosis. For these reasons we recommend you consult a nutrition counsellor (see How to Get Help).

In the meantime here are some simple steps anyone can take to promote and maintain mental and emotional health:

1 Avoid sugar and refined foods.

2 Eat more fresh fruit, vegetables and whole foods (e.g seeds, nuts, beans, lentils, wholegrains)

3 Reduce or avoid stimulants - namely tea, coffee, chocolate, cola drinks, cigarettes.

4 Reduce or avoid alcohol. The consumption of alcohol increases your allergic potential.

5 Cut down your 'pollution' load by reducing your time spent in smoky, high exhaust fume areas, and, if you smoke, stop smoking.

6 Have a heaped tablespoon of ground seeds (sesame, sunflower, pumpkin, flax), or a tablespoon of their oil every day.

7 If your diet contains a lot of wheat experiment with two weeks without it, eating oat cakes, rice cakes, corn or oat based cereals and buckwheat pasta instead. It is best to reintroduce a suspected allergen under the guidance of a nutritionist.

8 If your diet contains a lot of milk products (milk, cheese, yoghurt etc.) experiment with two weeks without milk products, using soya milk instead. It is best to reintroduce a suspected allergen under the guidance of a nutritionist.

Most habits take a month to break. So take one habit, like drinking coffee. Give yourself one month without it, then see how you feel. The healthier your diet the less will be the 'withdrawal' effects. The greater the withdrawal effects the worse this substance is for you. Take one step at a time and know that every step makes a difference.

Supplements for Mental Health

The brain uses about a third of all nutrients taken in from food. The following recommendations apply to anyone wishing to promote and maintain mental health.

1 Supplement your diet with a high strength multivitamin supplement containing vitamins A, D and E, plus C and B vitamins. Make sure your supplement contains at least 75mg of niacin, pantothenic acid (B5) and pyridoxine, and at least 100mcg of folic acid (unless you are histadelic and experiencing mental health problems) and 10mcg B12.

2 Supplement between 1,000mg and 3,000mg of vitamin C every day.

3 Supplement a high strength multimineral providing at least calcium 400mg, magnesium 200mg, zinc 15mg, manganese 5mg, chromium 100mcg, selenium 100mcg.

4 Unless you are eating seeds and/ or their oils most days consider supplementing Omega 6 oils, such as evening primrose or borage (sometimes known as starflower) oil and Omega 3 oils, from flaxseed (also known as linseed) or fish oils.

In addition you may choose to add the supplemental recommendations in chapters whose content specifically applied to you. Ensure that these recommended amounts of the specified nutrients are included in your daily supplement programme. See next page for a Directory of Supplement Companies. Wherever possible we recommend consutation with a qualified practitioner, who can run the appropriate tests, over self-supplementation.

DIRECTORY OF SUPPLEMENT COMPANIES

Bio Care produce a wide range of supplements available by mail-order. These include Chromium Polynicotinate, Bio-Magnesium, Zinc Citrate, Sucroguard, B-Plex (free from folic acid), Neurotone, Magnesium Taurate, Phosphatidyl Serine, Liquid Trace Minerals and others. Send for a free catalogue to: BioCare, Lakeside, 180 Lifford Lane, Kings Norton, Birmingham, B30 3NT. Tel: 0121 433 3727.

Health Plus produce an extensive range of supplements available by mail order including Multivitamin (free from folic acid), B6 + Zinc, Ziman Plus, B12 + Folic Acid, B3+Chromium, Evening Primrose Oil and others. Send for a free catalogue to: Health Plus Ltd, Dolphin House, 30 Lushington Road, Eastbourne, East Sussex, BN21 4LL Tel: 01323 737374.

Higher Nature produce an extensive range of supplements available by mail order including Brain Food with DMAE and Pyroglutamate, Chromium Polynicotinate, Hi-Phosphatidyl Choline, Glutamine powder, Niacin, Cal-M, Positive Nutrition - an amino acid complex for the brain, Starflower Oil, Flax Seed Oil and Essential Balance - a combination of organic cold-pressed oils. Send for a free catalogue to: Higher Nature, Burwash Common, East Sussex TN19 7LX Tel:01435 882880.

Lamberts produce an extensive range of supplements available to practitioners only. These include Phosphatidyl Choline, Glutathione Complex, B 50 Complex, Calcium Pantothenate, Pyridoxal -5-Phosphate, Folic Acid, Zinc Citrate, Manganese, L-Glutamine, Jay-Vee Tablets, DLPA Complex With Vitamins B and C, L-Methionine, Flax Seed Oil and others. Send for a free catalogue: Lamberts Healthcare Ltd., 1 Lamberts Road, Tunbridge Wells, Kent TN2 3EQ Tel: 01892 552121.

Solgar produce a wide range of supplements available from any good health food store. These include B complexes, B5, B6, Folate, Zinc, Manganese, Calcium, Magnesium + Zinc, Methionine, Neuro Nutrients, Phosphatidyl Serine, Gingko Biloba, No-Flush Niacin, Niacinamide, Lecithin, Phosphatidyl Choline and others. For your nearest stockist contact Solgar Vitamins Ltd, Chiltern Commerce Centre, Asheridge Road, Chesham, Buckinghamshire HP5 2PY Tel: 01494 791691.

USEFUL ADDRESSES

Carers National Association
20–25, Glasshouse Yard, London, EC1A 4JS   Tel: 0171 490 8818

Citizens Commission for Human Rights
PO Box 188, East Grinstead, West Sussex RH19 2FL Tel: 01622 726128

Hyperactive Children's Support Group
71 Whyke Lane, Chichester, West Sussex PO19 2LD.SAE please.

Institute for Optimum Nutrition
Blades Court, Deodar Road, London SW15 2NU   Tel: 0181 877 9993
ION offers courses and consultations with nutrition consultants, plus a
national directory of nutrition consultants (see page xx).

Laboratory tests are available for all the tests mentioned in this
book, through qualified nutrition consultants. Leading laboratories
include Biolab Medical Unit (doctors only) Tel: 0171 636 5959;
Diagnostech for adrenal stress testing Tel: 0121 458 3407; Immuno
Laboratories for IgG ELISA allergy testing Tel: 01435 882 880; and also
Larkhall Laboratories Tel: 0181 874 1130.

Manic Depression Fellowship 8–10 High Street,
Kingston–on–Thames, Surrey, KT1 1EY   Tel: 0181 974 6550

Mental Health Project
ION, Blades Court, Deodar Road, London SW15 2NU Tel: 0181 877
9993. Anyone can participate in this project by coming to meetings
advertised in ION's Optimum Nutrition magazine. The aim of the is to
put the message of this book into practice in the community.

MIND 22 Harley Street, London, W1N 2ED   Tel: 0181 519 2122

National Schizophrenia Fellowship 28 Castle Street,
Kingston–on–Thames, Surrey, KT1 1SS   Tel: 0181 547 3837

Natural Justice, The Gill, Ulverston,
Cumbria LA12 7BJ   Tel: 01229 5800555

Princeton Bio Center, 862 Route 518, Skillman,
New Jersey 08558, USA   Tel: 001 609 924 8607

SANE 199–205 Old Marylebone Road,
London, NW1 5QP   Tel: 0171 724 6520

Schizophrenia Association of Great Britain
Bryn Hyfryd, The Crescent, Bangor, Gwynnedd,
LL57 2AG   Tel: 01248 354048

RECOMMENDED READING

Optimum Nutrition
Patrick Holford, ION Press, 1994

Optimum Nutrition Workbook
Patrick Holford, ION Press, 1995

Mental Illness - Not All in the Mind
Edited by Patrick Holford, ION Press, 1995

The New Fatburner Diet
Patrick Holford, ION Press, 1995

Boost Your Immune System
Jennifer Meek, ION Press, 1996

Dr Braly's Food Allergy and Nutrition Revolution
Dr James Braly, Keats Publishing, 1992

Mental and Elemental Nutrients
Dr Carl Pfeiffer, Keats Publishing, 1975

Nutritional Influences on Mental Illness
Melvyn Werbach, 3rd Line Press, 1991

Smart Drugs and Nutrients
Ward Dean and John Morgenthaler, Health Freedom Publications, 1990

Vitamin B3 (Niacin), Dr Abram Hoffer, Keats, 1984

Vitamin B3 (Niacin) Update: New Roles for a Key Nutrient in Diabetes, Cancer, Heart Disease and Other Major Health Problems, Keats,1990

Smart Nutrients - A Guide to Nutrients That Can Prevent and Reverse Senility, Dr Abram Hoffer, Avery Publishing, 1994

Most of these books are available from the ION Bookclub, Blades Court, Deodar Road, London SW15 2NU. Please call 0181-871-4576 for a current price list.

References

Many references from respected scientific literature have been referred to in this book. A full list of these references, listed for each chapter, is available from the Institute for Optimum Nutrition, Blades Court, London SW15 2NU. Key references are numbered in the text. Please send £2 and an SAE. Most of these research papers can also be accessed at the Lamberts Library at ION. Please call 0181-877-9993 for details.

INDEX

Acetylcholine (see
neurotransmitters)
acetylcoenzyme A
(ACoA) 49,50
acne 128
addictions 53,162-167
additives 36, 42, 136
  as cause of hyperactivity 153,
  154
adrenals 58,130,133,134
adrenalin 57,95,96,116,130,133
alcohol 18, 60,64,73, 84,
97,104,107,110,119,130,133
alcoholism 139,165
allergies 61-67,139-141,
  cerebral 61,137
  cross reactions 66
  dairy 67
  delayed food sensitivities 61
  histamine and 136
  symptoms of 62
  testing 62-66,137-138
  wheat-gluten 136-8,143-144
aluminium 36,39-41,73,176
Alzheimers disease 39,69
amino acids 60
  cystine 42
  methionine 41
  tryptophan 95
  tyrosine 22
antibiotics 146
antihistamine 140
arsenic 41
arthritis 9
asthma 42,137
autism 145

Bipolar disorder 185
birth control pill 112
blood sugar levels
52,55,57,58,129,134
borage oil 34
brain development 15

cadmium 35,36,39-42, 92,127,158
calcium 23,41,51, 55,60,127,163,178-
182
  supplementation in histadelia
  103,106
cancer 10
carbohydrates 96,104,131
  complex 44,45,49,50,52,131,132
  refined 73
  simple 444,45,49,132
carbon dioxide 49
ceruloplasmin 110,112
chelators 40
chlorpromazine 191,193
chocolate 54,55,64,69,73,129
choline 60,69,71,182
chromium 18,49,51,60,131-133
coeliac disease 137
coenzyme Q 51,60
coffee 54,69,73,129,131
Cogentin 191
Colgan, Michael 72
colic 67
complex adaptive systems 11,12
copper 36,96,108,110-112,116,125-
127
Davies, Dr Stephen 40
dementia paralytica 101,113
depixol 184

depressants 60,93
depression 82,96,102,135,184
  and allergy 139
  manic 82,88,110
dermatitis 114
DGLA 28,34
DHA 31,32,68
DHEA 58
disperceptions 123
DMAE 69-71
dopamine excess 101
Downs syndrome 147
drug addiction 104
drug interactions 11
  side effects of 11,142,190-193
dyslexia 71,148,150

Ear infections 146
eczema 20,42,67
EDTA 40
EEG 37
EFA's (see fats-essential)
eicosapentaenoic acid 31
Einstein, Albert 9,10,13
endorphins 101
EPA 31,32,34,
epilepsy 24,128,182,183
evening primrose oil 31,34,149,
152,169

Fats 40,45,96
  essential 21,28,68,97,101,113,
  128,137
  saturated 28
  omega 3 28,32-34
  omega 6 28-34
folic acid (see Vitamin-folic acid)

GLA 29,163,175
Glucose 43-45,48,49,56,58,60
  level in blood 44,48
  tolerance factor (see GTF)
gluten 67,139-144
glycogen 44,45,58
GTF 45,46,58,129-134

Hemp 33
herbicides 35
heroine 162,166
herpes 128
histadelia 102107
  and drug addiction 164
histamine 64,77,95,102,108,
112,116,123
histapenia 101,108-112
histidine imbalance 101
Hoffer, Dr Abram 6,17,92,100,
113,115
homocystinuria 101
Huntingdon's chorea 101
hydrochloric acid 66
hyperactivity 137,149-155
hyperglycemia 46
hypoglycemia 101,129-134,157
hypothalamus 134
hypothyroidism 101

Ichazo, Oscar 59,
immunoglobulin 141,146
  IgE 61,62,64,65
  IgG 62-65
Institute for Optimum
Nutrition(see ION)
insomnia 179-181
insulin 45,46,57,7
ION 194,200,206

IQ studies 8,37,43,68-72
iron 51,54

Krebs cycle 50
Krehl, Dr 23
kryptopyrroles 118,
lactic acid 23,49
lactose 44
Lansdown, R 38
lead 9,35-40,42,73,92
lecithin 69,70
lithium 186-188

Magnesium 23,36,51,55,60,96,132,
146,150,159,163,180-183
manganese 18,21,24,60,108,111,
119,123,126,131-134,183,192,198
mauve factor 121
menstruation 185
mercury 36,39-42
methionine 103
milk allergy 144
mitochondria 49
monamine oxidase inhibitors 193
monopolar disorder 182

Narconon 162
Natural Justice 156
Needleman, Prof H 37
neurotransmitters 16,22,61,68, 91-
97,102,116
    acetylcholine 16,21,69-70,94,95
    adrenaline 95
    dopamine 95
    phenylalanine 95
    serotonin 16,95,101,116
Newton, Isaac 9
Niacin (see vitamin B3)

Niacinamide (see vitamin B3)
nicotine 166
nootropics 71

Oestrogen 38
Osmond, Dr Humphrey 17,155
oxygen 49

Parkinson's 95
Pasteur, Louis 9
pellagra 20,101,111-113
pesticides 3
Pfeiffer, Dr Carl 17,24,41,70,
76,77,80,92
Phenothiazines 25
phosphatidyl choline 71
phospholipids 68
phosphorus 41,132
Piracetam 71
porphyria 101
potassium 132
Princeton Bio Centre 17
prolactin excess 101
prostaglandin 29-31, 01,116,
Prozac 193
psoriasis 128
psychiatry 8
pyroglutamate 69,71,177
pyorrhoea 127
pyroluria 101,116-128
pyruvic acid 49,50

Quantum health 11
quanta 11,13
quarks 10

RDA 17,18,51,72,114,116
Recommended Daily Allowances
(see RDA)

Rimland, Dr Bernard 155
Ritalin 151,154
Rosenhan, Dr 11-13
Rudin, Donald 33

Schizophrenia
  causes of 94,110,115,135
  diagnosis of 80,82-86,89,98,100,
  105,113,118,131
  main types 88,97
seasonal affective disorder 186
seeds 34
selenium 39,41
senility 175-178
  aluminium linked 39
Serine excess 101
serotonin imbalance (see
neurotransmitters)
sleep deprivation 101
Sohler, Dr Arthur 25
SONAs 18
stress 56-60,84,119,121,127,133
  and caffeine 52,54,55,77
  and stimulants 48,49,53-60,69,
  93,129,130
  and theobromine 52,54
  and theophylline 52,54
sugar 52,55,56,73,90,93,104,
105,129,130
  in hypoglycemia 45,132
  sucrose 44

Tannin 54
tardive dyskinesia 30,190,192
tartrazine 36,42,136,153
tea 54
Thomas, Louise 33
tyrosine (see amino acids)

US National Research Council 25

Vanadium 186
Vitamin A 18
Vitamin B deficiency 20-22,26,51
  B2 50
  B6 (see pyridoxine)
  B12 17,21,22,50,101
  biotin 50
  folic acid 17,20-22,50,51,96,
  101,178,183
  niacin (B3) 17,20,21,31,50,96,
  111-117, 122, 150,153,163,165,
  176,178,182
  pantothenic acid (B5) 20,21,50,
  69,71,177,182
  pyridoxine (B6) 17,21,32,31,45,
  50,51,55,76,77,118,121-128,140,
  146,150,163,178,182,185
Vitamin C 17,18,22,23,36,40,41,
55,60,96,102,112,113,114,132,140,1
48,153,159,163,176,178,179
Vitamin E 18,192

Wheat-Gluten allergy 143-144
Wilson disease 101
Winneke, Dr G 38
World Health Organisation 30

Zinc 18,21,24,26,36,39-45,54,65,77,
90,108,111,118,121-129,134,136140,
146,148,150,159,163,169,173,174,1
78,179-181

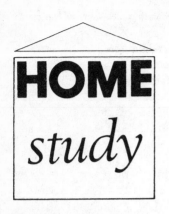

Your car comes with a manual, but what about your body?

What makes you tick? How do you make energy from food? Why do some people age faster - and how can you age more slowly? What's the secret for super-health?

You'll find many answers in **ION's Homestudy Course** (that comes with 3 workbooks, 3 hours of videos, 12 taped lectures and step by step instructions to give you a solid grounding in 10 weeks). You'll learn more than you thought possible and have fun doing it with practical homework and experiments.

Part 1 HOW YOUR BODY WORKS teaches you how to improve digestion and absorption, balance nerves and hormones, and boost immune power. The second part **FOOD & NUTRITION**, looks at everything from the politics of food to wholefood cookery. You'll find out how to prevent heart disease and protect against cancer and arthritis, as well as learning how to detect your own food intolerances. In the final part, **INDIVIDUAL NUTRITION**, you'll learn how to work out individually tailored programmes. You'll find out all about nutrition for children and the elderly, including nutritional 'first aid'.

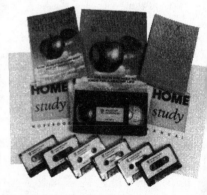

By the end of the course you'll know enough to keep yourself and your family healthy. When you enrol you'll get all the course materials, plus your own 'telephone tutor' to help you with any questions you have. Anyone can do it. All you need is a keen interest in nutrition.

Price: £150   **Members price: £135**

I O N

The Institute for Optimum Nutrition is a non profit-making independent organisation that exists to help you promote your health through nutrition. ION was founded in 1984 and is based in London. ION offers educational courses starting with a one-day introductory course right up to a three year training to become a nutrition consultant; a clinic for one-to-one consultations; publications and ION's magazine, Optimum Nutrition, which goes out free to members. If you'd like to receive more details please complete the details below.

Please send me your:

☐ FREE Information Pack on all ION services
☐ FREE BookClub Bulletin
☐ Directory of Nutrition Consultants
(enclose £2 plus A5 SAE)

I'd like to order the following books: *(please list title, quantity & price)*

_____

_____

_____

I enclose £ _____ payable to ION (Please add 10% for p&p)

First Name: _____ Surname: _____

Address: _____

_____ Postcode: _____

Now send this to: ION, Blades Court, Deodar Road,
London SW15 2NU (Tel: 0181 877 9993)

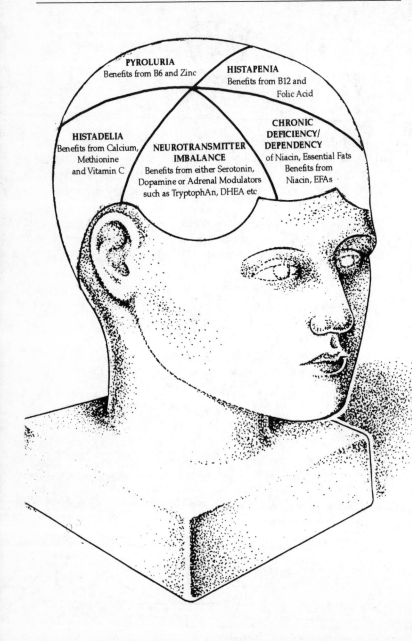

PYROLURIA
Benefits from B6 and Zinc

HISTAPENIA
Benefits from B12 and
Folic Acid

HISTADELIA
Benefits from Calcium,
Methionine
and Vitamin C

NEUROTRANSMITTER
IMBALANCE
Benefits from either Serotonin,
Dopamine or Adrenal Modulators
such as TryptophAn, DHEA etc

CHRONIC
DEFICIENCY/
DEPENDENCY
of Niacin, Essential Fats
Benefits from
Niacin, EFAs